PICTORIAL HISTORY

OF

ANCIENT PHARMACY;

WITH

𝔖𝔨𝔢𝔱𝔠𝔥𝔢𝔰 of 𝔈𝔞𝔯𝔩𝔶 𝔐𝔢𝔡𝔦𝔠𝔞𝔩 𝔓𝔯𝔞𝔠𝔱𝔦𝔠𝔢.

BY HERMANN PETERS.

TRANSLATED FROM THE GERMAN, AND REVISED, WITH NUMEROUS
ADDITIONS,

BY DR. WILLIAM NETTER.

SECOND EDITION.

Preface.

THE original work of Mr. Hermann Peters was a pioneer pathbreaker in even the prolific German historical field. It was an outgrowth of Mr. Peters' studies in the Germanic Museum at Nuremburg, and was pervaded by zeal for the reputation of the old city. This gave the style of the work a quaint fascination, which greatly increased its value in Germany, where intense interest is felt concerning Nuremburg, where so much of Germany's art, science, mechanical art and literature were fostered. The prominence of this quaint Nuremburgian patriotism in the work, while not without its charm, was a serious limitation and defect in a work intended for an English-speaking public.

The revision has therefore introduced many features of especial interest to English-speaking pharmacists and physicians, while retaining for the most part the style, arrangement and illustrations of the original.

The development of Pharmacy as a specialty of Medicine has been more carefully discussed in the light of researches not pursued by Mr. Peters. The original chapter on "Pharmacy in the Middle Ages" has been rewritten from the standpoint of the researches of Gordon, Baas, Hallam and Meryon. The chapter on "Ancient Pharmacopœias" and that on the "Development and Decline of Alchemy" have been considerably amplified, the former being supplemented by the results of the researches of Dr. Charles Rice, of New York, and other authorities.

The additions on the subject of American pharmacy are by Dr. James G. Kiernan, to whom the editor is indebted for much assistance in all original portions of the work.   W. N.

Illustrations.

(vii)

Contents.

CHAPTER III.

PHARMACY IN THE SIXTEENTH CENTURY.

CHAPTER IV.

PHARMACY IN THE SEVENTEENTH CENTURY.

CHAPTER V.

PHARMACY IN THE EIGHTEENTH CENTURY.

CHAPTER VI.

DISTILLING APPARATUS.

CHAPTER VII.

EARLY CHEMICO-PHARMACAL STOVES AND FIRE-PLACES.

CHAPTER VIII.

ANCIENT PHARMACOPŒIAS.

CHAPTER IX.

MEDICAL SUPERSTITIONS.

CHAPTER X.

PHARMACY AND THE ART OF LOVE.

CHAPTER XI.

ALCHEMY.

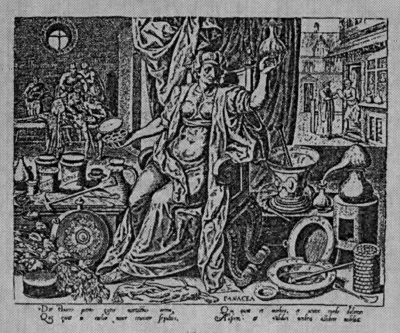

Fig. 2.

MEDICINE, PHARMACY AND SURGERY.
(An allegorical representation of the Sixteenth Century).

I, Apollo, the science of all herbs have conceived ;
  To me are their virtues and powers revealed.
Thus " Master of Art " bv me was received.
  A title mine own by eternity sealed.

—HIERONYMUS BOCK.
(Book of Herbs, 1551.)

CHAPTER X.

PHARMACY AND THE ART OF LOVE.

CHAPTER XI.

ALCHEMY.

Tutelar Gods and Patron Saints of Medicine and Pharmacy.

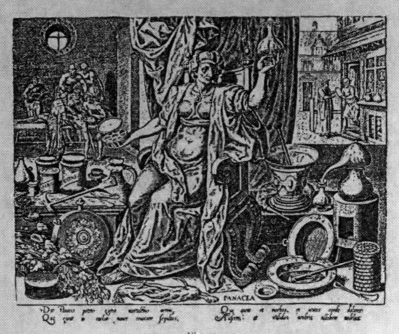

Fig. 2.

MEDICINE, PHARMACY AND SURGERY.
(An allegorical representation of the Sixteenth Century).

Chapter One.

Tutelar Gods and Patron Saints of Medicine and Pharmacy.

CY and medicine in most countries had
ion origin in the fetichtic philosophy of the
which recognized a "soul" in even inani-
bjects. Disease was the "soul" of one
object attacking another, and to drive this malign
influence off, noises, smells, and various contortions were employed, such as are still used by the "medicine men" of the
savages of to-day. The fact was empirically ascertained that
herbs* had beneficent properties which were at first explained on
the fetichtic philosophy. On this double basis of empiricism
and a fanciful philosophy developed pharmacy, medicine, and
most religions.

For a long period the religious incantations formed the chief
part in the treatment of disease. The chanter of litanies occupied a higher place than the physician who applied the remedies.
This relationship was later removed. The cuneiform inscriptions in Assyria contain a complete history of this evolution.
The earlier inscriptions give a prominent place to charms and
incantations in medicine. The later (B. C. 1640) contain
reference to classified diseases, their pathology, diagnosis and
treatment, including directions for the preparation of medicine.
One inscription, for example, directs the preparation of a prescription for a "diseased gall bladder which devours the top of
a man's heart; cypress extract, goat's milk, palm wine, barley,
ox and bear flesh, and the wine of the cellarer,"† are directed to

* Schultze, History of Fetichism.
† Sayce, "Translations of the Cuneiform Inscriptions."

be made into a decoction by a medical specialist clearly practicing pharmacy.

The researches of Ebers leave little doubt that pharmacy was practiced by one branch of the priesthood of Isis, to whom prescriptions were sent by the physician-priest, who, accompanied by a chanter of litanies or charms, attended the sick.

Some of the Egyptian inscriptions indicate that processes akin to distilling were practiced.* How far these influenced the later discoveries of the Arabian chemists is an open question, since it is well known that the alleged destruction of the Alexandrian library is a myth.

The Aryan† races had similar usages to the Assyrians in regard to the commingling of religion, pharmacy, and medicine. Chinese pharmacy and pathology is a corrupted form of the earlier Aryan views.

Fig. 3.
ISIS.

One Aryan expression of the indignation of the priests at the increasing tendency to the separation of medicine and science from religion was to be found in the Greek myth of Prometheus. When Prometheus, an early friend of man, had wrenched fire from the hands of Zeus, and presented it to the poor mortals, the wrath of the king of the gods knew no bounds, and he determined upon being revenged. Pursuant to this he ordered Hephæstos to model a woman, and induced all the immortal gods to adorn her with the costliest gifts at their command. The result was a being of resplendent and fascinating loveliness, named Pandora. To Hermes fell the lot of conducting her to the earth and into the presence of Epimetheus. Although forewarned by his brother Prometheus, not to accept presents from Zeus, Epimetheus nevertheless could not withstand the beauty and attractiveness of Pandora, giving her hospitable shelter and accepting from her a box as a gift from the gods. Hardly had he lifted the lid when there poured forth from the box wailings and lament, hunger and want, distress, sickness and

* Zeitschrift für Egyptologie, 1865.
† History of Medicine, by Gordon.

suffering immeasurable. Becoming terrified and quickly attempting to close the box, he saw that Hope, which was the last to leave the box, had been caught by the lid, and thus the only consoler of man ever afterward presented itself to him in a sadly distorted condition. Ever since this occurrence wasting fevers haunt the land, and pale and hollow-eyed disease pursues man wherever he goes. But Prometheus, by order of Zeus, was chained to the most desolate rock in the Caucasus.

The myth further tells us that a certain god took pity on suffering man, and, in a measure at least, to console and help him, taught him the art of healing. This god was Æsculapius. According to the legend, he was the son of Hermes and Caronis, was born in the neighborhood of Epidaurus, and was there left to his fate at the foot of a mountain. A goat there nourished him, and a shepherd dog protected and watched over him. Later on Hermes intrusted his education to the Centaur Chiron, who mainly instructed him in the art of healing. Æsculapius was an apt scholar, and very soon became such a master in the art that he not only healed the sick and wounded, but even brought the dead to life again. This restoration of the dead excited the wrath of Pluto, the god of Hades, who complained to Zeus, and the latter killed the culprit with a thunderbolt for daring to interfere with the natural limits of human life.

Another later legend assigns as the real cause of his sudden and ignoble taking off, that he had, contrary to the will of the gods, taught the art of healing to man. The grateful mortals did not forget their benefactor, and built temples in honor of Æsculapius, in which priests, of whom his two sons, Podalirius and Machaon, were the first in order, further practiced and developed the art of healing. Æsculapius is pictured as a most worthy and wise-looking, long-bearded man, bearing in his hand a staff around which coiled a snake. The preparing of the medicine ordered was left to Hygeia, the goddess of healing, who was the daughter, or, according to others, the wife of Æsculapius.

Thus modern healers, whose path in life is not always strewn with roses, and whose efforts in behalf of suffering man are frequently no more appreciated than were those of Æsculapius of old by the gods, may look to this patron saint for consolation, and furthermore take pride in the charming Hygeia, who is portrayed as a youthful and beautiful woman, clad in a long flowing robe, in the act of feeding a serpent from a shell.

In the medical works of the Romans, Greeks, and those of the Middle Ages, these gods of healing are frequently referred

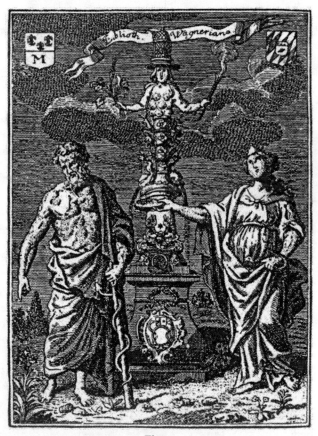

Fig. 4.

ÆSCULAPIUS AND HYGEIA.

(From a plate of the Eighteenth Century).

to. Figure 4 represents these two gods. It is a reproduction from a copper-plate executed by J. P. Funk, of Nuremburg, in the eighteenth century. The picture bearing the inscription, "Bibliotheca Wagneriana," served as a property mark in a

"Fauna suecica Carol. Linnæi," still preserved in the Germanic museum. Whether or not the former owner of the book is identical with his namesake, the noted Famulus in Goethe's Faust, we must leave undecided. But the portrayal of nature between

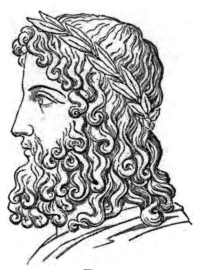

Fig. 5.

ÆSCULAPIUS.

the figures of Æsculapius and Hygeia at least vividly calls to mind these words of Faust, rendered by Bayard Taylor :

"How grand a show ! but ah ! a show alone.
Thou boundless nature, how make thee my own ?
Where you, ye breasts ?   Founts of all Being, shining,
Whereon hang Heaven's and Earth's desire,
Whereto our withered hearts aspire,—
Ye flow, ye feed ; and am I vainly pining ?"

Although in the original myth Prometheus and Æsculapius appear as enemies to the priesthood, who believed in the fetichtic doctrine of the origin of disease, the worship of the latter as a subsidiary god soon became fashionable, while the observations of Hippocrates and Galen, and the researches of the Athens Archæological Society* show that the temples of Æsculapius and

* Kumanudes, Athenaion; Corpus Inscriptionum Atticarum.

Hygiea were in reality hospitals attended by skilled physicians. The cure or improvement of the patient was ascribed to the power of the god or goddess invoked by the worship or offerings of the patient. Treatment was often indicated by the god, in a vision, to the physician. Hippocrates, whose family had been priests of Æscupalius at Cos, directs physicians to pay particular attention to the dreams of the patient and himself.

Fetichism rapidly passed into pure symbolism, and the principle of life and health was early represented as a serpent, whose graceful, stealthy motion had early excited curiosity. In many of the Egyptian incantations for health this serpent worship played a part. On one notable occasion Moses and the Hebrews are found returning to this worship. The symbol early and naturally became a medical one, and associated with Æsculapius and Hygiea.* Around the staff of Æsculapius a serpent winds, and the assumption of this staff by an ordained priest was celebrated by an annual festival.†

When the intellectual revolution produced by the teachings of Christ swept over the world the old gods and goddesses were replaced by Christian saints. In Greece, in the places formerly sacred to Hygeia, the Virgin is invoked to cure disease.‡ In Western Europe the holy martyrs, Cosmas and Damian, took the place of Æsculapius in popular worship, and their portraits were henceforth frequently placed on the title pages of medical works. The two saints, who were brothers, lived in the fourth century. Deeply moved by the Christian religion, they were actuated by the noblest motives, and practiced the art of healing with the utmost self-sacrifice. When the Diocletian persecution of Christians was inaugurated, they were arrested by order of the city's mayor, Lysias, and condemned to death. The legend says that during their execution and shortly thereafter, a number of miracles took place. In a book entitled "The Holy Lives," printed by Martin Hupfuf, in the free and imperial city of Strassburg in 1513, it is related that when the saints had been thrown into the water with the purpose of drowning them, an angel descended, and, freeing their bounden limbs, enabled them to gain the shore. Lysias then ordered them to be burned,

* Schultze, History of Fetichism.
† Littre, Vol. IV.
‡ Merriam. Trans. N. Y. Academy of Medicine, 1886.

but the fire attacked the heathen and many of them perished. They were then fastened to a cross, and Lysias ordered them to be stoned to death and pierced by arrows; but in each instance these missiles proved to be boomerangs in the hands of the would-be slayers. Becoming very much enraged at these futile attempts, he had them beheaded, whereupon their souls took flight heavenward. Their bodies were taken to Asyria and preserved in a chapel. Pope Felix procured some of their relics, which he placed in a church built in honor of the two saints.

For centuries physicians and patients journeyed to the shrine of the saintly patrons of medicine, and many patients were reported to have been healed. One instance of miraculous healing should here be recorded. A man with a diseased leg had fervently implored them to come to his relief in his great suffering, and his faith in the supernatural powers ascribed to them was soon to be rewarded. One night he dreamed that they were in his presence, and were holding counsel over his stricken member. They concluded to replace it by a sound limb taken from a Moor who had but recently died. When he awoke the new member was in place, and at once served the purpose of a useful limb, causing amazement among the populace, and serving to confirm their belief in the superhuman powers of the saints.

To the fact that the limb of a Moor had served to perform this miracle, as well as to the profound impression the occurrence left upon the minds of men, is probably due the predilection that so many druggists of the Middle Ages displayed toward the sign of the Moor, which was by them so frequently chosen as a badge or emblem, to which peculiarity, even at the present day, the many "Apotheken zum Mohren" in Central Europe bear witness. In many parts of Europe the 27th day of September, the day of martyrdom of these Catholic Christian saints, was celebrated in a pompous manner. The Vienna Medical Society possesses a copy of an invitation, in Latin, of the year 1700, in which physicians, licentiates, baccalaureates, students, druggists and surgeons are invited to take part in a grand celebration of the Cosmas and Damian anniversary in the Stephans church at Vienna.

Very likely the pictures of the saints were on such occasions multiplied and distributed among the populace, as is done at the present time when a nation honors its heroes. The Vienna

Medical Society also possesses two copper-plates that evidently served this purpose. Figure 6 is reproduced from one of these plates.

Figure 2, which introduces this chapter, represents the art of healing, with its sub-divisions, Medicine, Pharmacy and Surgery,

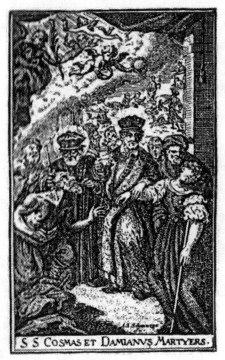

S. S. COSMAS ET DAMIANUS MARTYRES.

Fig. 6.
COSMAS AND DAMIANUS.

It is from a copper-plate by an unknown master of the sixteenth century. In the background a drug store stands revealed by the peculiar bottles and containers displayed in the windows, and a druggist appears at the door of his shop in plain garb, humbly accepting a prescription from the hands of the physician. Pharmacy is further represented by a mortar and distilling apparatus, as well as by numerous roots and herbs promiscuously distributed in the foreground.

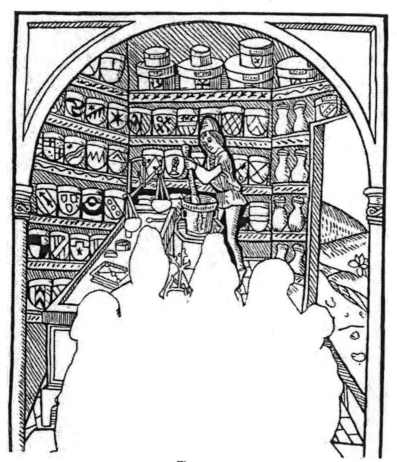

Fig. 7.

(From a book of 1486).

Noting his penury to myself I said :
And if a man did need a poison now,
Whose sale is present death in Mantua,
Here lives a caitiff wretch would sell it him.

—ROMEO AND JULIET.

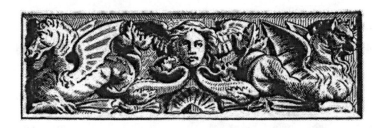

Chapter Two.

Pharmacy in the Middle Ages.

HARMACY early attained a relatively high development among the Egyptians. A papyrus of the
reign of Sent (3300 years B. C.) gives directions as
to the preparation of prescriptions. These were
given accompanied by incantations. By 1600 B. C.
medicine and pharmacy were as far advanced among the Egyptians as at the time of Galen Claudius (200 A. D.) In the Ebers
papyri (1600 B. C.) is a formulary containing prescriptions of
famous physicians. Among these are several of a noted Assyrian
ophthalmologist living near Mt. Lebanon. Draughts, blisters,
powders, ointments, and clysters are the chief preparations mentioned. Mineral and vegetable drugs are used. That the " art of
the apothecary," however, already existed among Assyrians
is shown by these prescriptions, as well as the inscriptions in
cuneiform letters* which give formulæ for various diseases.

The Hebrews, from their association with the Egyptians and
the Assyrians, imbibed a taste for pharmacal and medical
studies, and the " art of the apothecary " is spoken of very early
in Old Testament history. This bias the Hebrews never lost.
They had a medical school of their own at Sora as late as
200 A. D.

The influence of the Cushito-Aryan civilization, which showed
itself in the wisdom of the Assyrians, left an impress on Central
Asia evident in the early development of pharmacy and medicine
among the Chinese, for Ching Nong, a contemporary of Menes I,
of Egypt, was learned in pharmacy. He studied botany and made

---

* Sayce. (15)

decoctions and extracts.   The Chinese drug-stores of to-day give
an idea of pharmacy as practiced for centuries among these
people.

Nearly all of the medicines, with a few important exceptions,
consist of nuts, berries, roots, barks, and herbs.   The subjoined
list, furnished by a Chinese physician in Philadelphia, gives some
idea of the substances actually employed in practice :

正防主   Chiṅg fong tong.   The root of a plant.

何首烏   Ho Shau U.   Root of Aconitum Japonicum.

鮮髮乂   Tai tong kwai.   Root of Aralia edulis.

此菜杞   Hung kwo ki.   Fruit of wild Berberis Lycium.

壯粱   Pak'kí.   A kind of lung wort.

司芎   Ch'ün kung.   "Nodular masses, consisting apparently of the root-stock of some umbelliferous plant allied to
angelica."

甘草   Kòm ts'ò.   Liquorice root.

淮山   Wái shán.   The root of a water plant.

白茂   Pák shut.   The root of Atractylodes alba.

The herbs and barks are in large pieces, and the tubers and
roots usually entire.   It is customary to cut the former in small
pieces, and slice the latter in delicate segments before placing
them in the drawers and boxes for sale.   A large cleaver (yeúk
ts'oi k'ap), mounted with a hinge upon a slightly inclined table,
is employed to chop the grasses and herbs in convenient lengths,
while the tubers are sliced upon an instrument resembling a
carpenter's plane (yéuk p'ò), inserted in a long bench upon which
the operator sits, the pieces falling through upon a tray placed
beneath.   A canoe-shaped cast-iron mortar (yeúk shün) is employed to reduce some nuts and minerals to powder.   It stands
upon four legs, and a heavy iron disc is rolled backwards and
forwards within it by means of a wooden axle, to which the
operator applies his feet, while his hands are free to perform
other work.

The prescriptions furnished by the native doctors, which are
usually written upon Chinese letter paper, and a foot in length,
contain only a list of the names and quantities of the medicines
required, with concise directions for their preparation, no date

or signature being appended. The clerk weighs out the ingredients, and places them separately upon a large sheet of paper, going over them carefully afterward to prevent any possible mistake. A hand balance (litang) is used, consisting of a decimally graduated, ivory rod, from one end of which a brass scale pan is suspended by silk threads. The smaller kind weigh from one lf to five and one-half léung, or Chinese ounces, and are remarkably accurate. Some are powdered in the upright iron mortar (chung hòm), and others in the porcelain mortar (lúi ún); certain roots and seeds are roasted in a pan, while others are steeped for a few moments in Chinese rice spirits. The package of medicine is carried home to be boiled, and the infusion taken at one dose by the patient. Some Chinese prunes (hak tsò) are usually furnished, to be eaten at the same time. The prescription, of which no record is kept, is returned with the medicine.

The extensive materia medica of the Aryans* and the Sanscrit code of ethics show that the apothecary's art was in high esteem. The doctrine of transmigration of souls, as it limited the field of surgery, gave increased importance to pharmacology, botany and the preparation of drugs. The Greeks, from an early period, like most Aryan people, had a tinge of pharmacal knowledge, shown by the instruction given by the Centaurs (symbols of foreign influence) to the various gods and heroes. Pharmacy among the Greeks was stimulated by the necessity of additions to the incantations of the priests. The mixed religious and medical procedures in the marvels recorded in the temples of Hygiea and Æsculapius indicate this.

An additional stimulus was given by the use of a poison by the state for public executions, and the necessity the fair sex felt of adding to their attractions. A poem of Theocritus ("Pharmaceutica") deals chiefly with philters, then a profitable branch of pharmacy, which, even to the present day, survives in the "love powders," so largely in demand in certain districts of our larger cities.

In the temples of Æsculapius the art of medicine became somewhat systematized; pharmacists resided within the walls, while the physicians went forth among the people. This is obvious from many of the facts cited by Hippocrates (B. C. 460–

* Gordon, History of Medicine.

370), who gathered up many of the observations recorded by his predecessors. He was the seventh of seven of the same name, and the most illustrious of a long line of medical men. Pharmacy and medicine, which had begun to diverge under the Æsclepiades, became united in his person. Hippocrates carried his drugs with him.

Greek and Egyptian medicine and pharmacy commingled at Alexandria, where every science of the period was stimulated by the Ptolemies (323–30 B. C.) Among the great pharmacists and

Fig. 8.

HIPPOCRATES.

physicians of this period were : Herophilos (335 B. C.), who made great contributions to anatomy. He also made several contributions to pharmacology. Serapion (280 B. C.) and Mantias (250 B. C.) wrote formularies giving descriptions of drugs and processes; Herakleides added much to the pharmacology of Hippocrates; Appollonios, of Tyre, and Dioscorides, of Phakas, were toxicologists, pharmacologists and magicians ;* Erasistratos was the great anatomist of the period.

By the empirical school, which developed under the teachings of Herophilos and Erasistratos (280 B. C.), pharmacology and therapeutics were greatly studied. Through the experiments on human beings of Mithridates and Attalos III, toxicology

* Baas, "Geschichte der Medicin."

received an impetus. The cosmetic art was advanced by Cleopatra, by Berenice and Arsenœa, who dabbled in this branch of the pharmacy of the period. Kleophantos (138 B. C.), Nikandros (136 B. C.), Kratenos (70 B. C.) and Heras (30 B. C.), contributed much to pharmacology.

The early Roman writings on medicine discuss hygiene and preventive medicine. Vegetius (386 B. C.) wrote a work on the duties of army surgeons, which pays but little attention to pharmacy. His directions, where not surgical, are chiefly dietetic and hygienic.

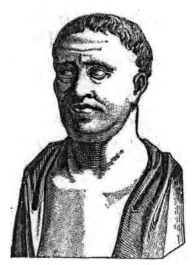

Fig. 9.

ÆSCLEPIADES.

About 187 B. C., in consequence of an epidemic, a temple was erected to Æsculapius, and later one to Hygiea. This introduced pharmacy and therapeutics into Rome. About 100 B. C., Arcagathus left Greece for Rome, and a "shop and surgery" were purchased for him by the people. He practiced both medicine and pharmacy. He was driven out on account of his predilection for operations, and was succeeded in popular esteem by Æsclepiades, who had studied medicine at Alexandria, then the great centre of Græco-Egyptian medicine. He practiced an expectant treatment and hydropathy, and denounced drugs and venesection. Themiston, who was practically his pupil, suc-ceeded him. Medicine soon became divided up into sects and specialties. The tendency to pharmacy was shown in the extensive use of drugs by some of these sects, who acquired a peculiar skill in dispensing.* Menecrates (1 A. D.) was one of these. He invented diachylon plaster, and used it for much the same purposes for which it is employed to-day. Archigenes, who was his successor, employed opium in dysentery.

Fig. 10.

GALEN.

Dioscorides, of Anazarba, who belonged to the Græco-Roman school of this period, was a great pioneer in pharmacy. He extended the knowledge of botany and pharmacology in a work which was recognized as an authority on the subject as late as the seventeenth century, A. D. Dioscorides used powdered elm-bark in skin diseases, and polypodium as an anthelmintic. He described four hundred plants. His followers in pharmacology were Varro (27 B. C.) and Macersen. Celsus was a commentator rather than a pharmacist or physician.

* Gordon.

Galen, the great reviver of medicine, who maintained his supremacy for nearly fourteen hundred years, was at once pharmacist, physician, botanist and surgeon. He united in his works the various schools. He is on record as keeping a drug store in Rome. His theories as to disease still in small degree dominate modern pathology. In many particulars he reproduced the theories of the Aryan physicians, and that school of Aryan medicine which prevailed in China. He was the first to secure the aroma of plants by distillation. To the list of plants given by Dioscorides he added nearly half as many more. One class of remedies described by him were called "Arteriacea," which acted on the blood vessels in a similar manner to the "vasomotor" remedies of to-day.

In the next century appear three great names, Ruffus, who discovered the function of the recurrent laryngeal nerve, Aurelianus, and Leonidas. Isolation of contagious diseases was proposed by Aurelianus and Leonidas, who were denounced by the public as brutes for so doing. The next two centuries were periods of decline. Nemesius, in his work "De Natura Hominis" (300 A.D.), gives a theory of the circulation of the blood, which, imperfect though it be, is a step forward in the direction of the modern doctrine. Oribasius, in the fourth century, was an active pharmacologist. Ætius, in the fifth century, first made use of the magnet in the treatment of disease.

Alexander Trallianus, in the sixth century, advised that age, sex, and constitution be considered in treatment. He used colchicum in the treatment of gout, iron in the treatment of anæmia, rhubarb in "liver weakness" and dysentery. He introduced the mixture called "hiera picra" into medicine as an anthelmintic. He distinguished between tape-worms, round worms, and thread worms. In the sixth century, Pope Gregory the Great enunciated the dogma of Homœopathy, which had been propounded in China several centuries before.* Paulus Ægineta, in the seventh century, described Chinese rhubarb. As early as the second century a Jewish University existed at Sora, where medicine was taught.

With the rise of the Saracens into intellectual dominance, the

* Meryon, p. 115.

Græco-Roman, Græco-Egyptian, and Cushito-Aryan schools of medicine and pharmacy became united.

The practitioners of medicine were held in high esteem by the Arabians. Mahomet himself had a predilection for the healing art. There is very good reason for believing that numerous medical works were preserved from the destruction of the Alexandrian library, by the Arabian physicians. It is certain that the Arabs had medical schools at Alexandria for more than a century after the alleged destruction of the library.

The practice of pharmacy was greatly extended by the Arabians, and among them the separation of medicine and pharmacy was recognizable as early as the eighth century, and was established by law in the eleventh. There were two great schools among them. One held the view enunciated by Alkekendi in the ninth century, that "the activity of a medicine increases in a duplicate ratio when compounded with others," and were polypharmacists. The other school, noticeably Avicenna, opposed this view, which finally received its *coup de grace* at the hands of Averroes in the twelfth century.

As many of the drugs used were imported from the East, a branch of dealers sprung up who were to be distinguished from the apothecaries. These were, properly speaking, physicians who practiced pharmacy, and who existed in Italy as early as the eleventh century. The school of Salerno compelled its graduates* to swear not to give or accept percentages on prescriptions. This school was founded in the seventh century, and subsequently came under the control of the Arabs, and adopted from them the practice of separating medicine from pharmacy. Arctuarius, who wrote in the eleventh century, discusses pharmacy at great length. He describes laxatives in an exhaustive manner, and discusses "distilled waters." It is certain that establishments for dispensing medicines existed at Cordova, Toledo, and other large towns under the dominion of the Arabs, prior to the twelfth century, and establishments of this character were placed under severe legal restrictions. From their regulation Emperor Frederic II drew the material for the law passed in 1233 (which remained in force for a long

* Meryon.

time in the Two Sicilies), for the regulation of the practice of pharmacy.*

According to this law every medical man was required to give information against any pharmacist who should sell bad medicine. Pharmacists were divided into two classes. First, the *stationarii*, who sold simple medicines and "*non-magistral*" preparations, according to a tariff determined by competent authorities; and, second, the *confectionarii*, whose business consisted in scrupulously dispensing the prescriptions of the medical men. All pharmacal establishments were placed under the surveillance of the College of Medicine.

During the Middle Ages pharmacy was, to a great extent, under control of the Arabian physicians. From contact with them in the East, the religious orders (the Benedictines particularly) devoted themselves to pharmacy, pharmacology and therapeutics. These monks were forbidden to shed blood, with the result that surgery fell largely into the hands of the barbers. In the twelfth century the Benedictine monk, Ægidus, wrote a poetical treatise on drugs, which was long accepted by the schools as an authority. The rise of alchemy, the toxicological studies which the fashion of the age cultivated, and the taste for spices, combined medicine, pharmacy, chemistry, toxicology, the grocery business, the confectionery business and barbering into one trade, which united the learned with the criminal poisoner.

Under the auspices of the Saracens, pharmacy attained in Spain and Italy a status it never lost. The development of national life in Germany and England having taken place somewhat later than in other parts of Europe, the beginning of pharmacal history in the former is of a comparatively recent date. The cities give the earliest manifestations of the division of labor in medicine, which signalizes the origin of independent pharmacy.

In Germany the history of pharmacy begins in the thirteenth century. In 1267 a drug-store is found to exist at Muenster, in 1285 one at Augsburg, and in 1318 still another one at Hildesheim. The latter was originally the property of the church, but

* Hoefer, Histoire de la Chimie depuis les Temps les plus reculés jusqu'a notre Epoque, 1842.

after the year 1365 was controlled by the city. Undoubtedly other large German cities had drug-stores at this time, although definite records are not extant. That the boundary line of medicine and pharmacy was even then (1350) clearly defined is proven by the existence of a parchment ordinance of the city of Nuremberg. This decree ordains that the druggist shall conscientiously fill all written and verbal orders on him according to his best ability ; that he shall use none but pure drugs ; that he shall treat rich and poor with equal courtesy ; that he shall be modest in his charges, and not demand more than he needs to feed and clothe himself and those dependent upon him, allowing a reasonable advance on the price of the drug as a compensation for his services.

In those early days medicinal substances were largely imported from Italy. The remainder consisted in great part of simple mechanical mixtures and compounds. From these facts it is evident that these early drug-stores partook largely of the character of grocery stores. They were, in fact, a survival of the stationarii of the edict of 1233. In France and England grocers and spicers were early united with apothecaries. There was, however, not a little internecine contest between the mere drug and spice seller and the practitioner of pharmacy. The first considered himself only a merchant ; the latter affiliated with the physicians and surgeons. This internecine strife led to a separation, to the great discomfiture of the grocers, who were thus deprived of the profits arising from the sale of "strong waters."

In 1345 King Edward III of England gave a pension of of six pence a day to Coursus de Gangland, an apothecary of London, for taking care of and attending his majesty during his illness in Scotland. That the separation of the apothecary from the physician was pretty complete about this time, and that the populace suspected both of giving and taking percentages on prescriptions, will appear from the "Canterbury Tales," in which Chaucer says about his physician :

> " Full ready had he apotecaries
> To send him drugs and lectuaries,
> For each of them made other to winne
> Their friendship was not new to begin."

The grocers and apothecaries were legally united in England at this time by act of Parliament.

The first trace of a pharmacal corporate body is to be found in Bruges, in Belgium, in 1297. This corporation possessed at the beginning of the fourteenth century a spacious hall for its affairs, a seal, statutes, and a chapel. Here divine service was daily performed, new members were admitted and sworn in. Besides other wares, they had the exclusive sale of medicines. Members of distinguished families belonged to the guild, held the office of magistrate and other positions of dignity. The corporation, being possessed of great riches and privileges, gave the town at different times large sums for patriotic purposes. Our earliest knowledge of ancient established pharmacies we owe to wood-cuts coeval with the early human exploits in fields of science which collectively form the early chapters of a history of civilization. The wood-cut of those olden days frequently imparts clearer ideas concerning the pharmacist's life than words could convey. Bruges is known to have had its apothecaries from the earliest days of the fourteenth century. The first recorded apothecary shop in London was mentioned in 1345, the first in France in 1336, the first in Germany in the thirteenth century.

A very ancient memorial of an apothecaries guild, Fig. 11, may be seen in the gateway of the Minster at Ulm (Germany). It is an epitaph with the picture of a woman in the civilian dress of the fourteenth century. She is seen standing on a dog, with her head resting on a pillow, which bears the coat of arms of the "Ehinger" family. The inscription on the margins of the stone reads as follows: "In 1383. died. margareta. hainczen winkel's daughter. apothecaress. On saint Mathews' day." The presence of the "Ehinger" coat of arms lends plausibility to the inference that the husband of the "apothecaress," "whose family name is not given," was a member of the Ehinger family. The dog under the female figure (frequently pictured in this position on the epitaph of the female dead in the Middle Ages) denotes that the soul of the departed has now surmounted all carnal and earthly desires. During the Middle Ages and in antiquity the dog was looked upon not as a symbol of faithfulness, but as an unclean animal.

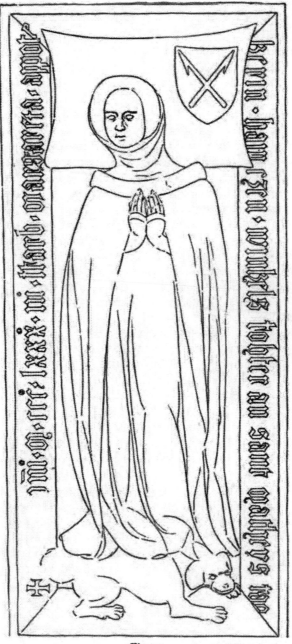

Fig. 11.
MEMORIAL OF THE APOTHECARIES GUILD AT ULM, A. D. 1380.

(26)

Figure 12, probably the oldest illustration of a drug-store extant, is taken from the "Ars Memorativa," published by Anton Sorg in 1470. Its most salient feature is a druggist comminuting some drug in a three-legged mortar. Before the introduction of chemistry into pharmacy the mortar was no doubt the pharmacist's principal companion, for the breaking up of crude drugs was then his main pharmacal manipulation. The back-

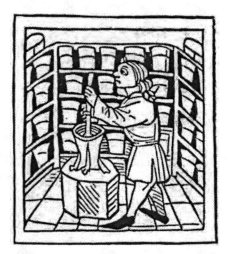

Fig. 12.
ILLUSTRATION OF DRUG-STORE, 1450.

ground is taken up by shelves that are loaded down with containers from floor to ceiling.

Figure 7, which introduces this chapter, taken from the work "Ortus sanitatis" (the "Garden of Health"), represents a drug-store. At the end of the book are these words: "Gedruckt vnd volendet diser Herbarius durch Hannsen schönsperger in der Keserylichen statt zu Augspurg an sant Bonifacius tag Anno MCCCC vn in dem LXXXVI jare." [This herbarium was printed and completed by Hannsen Schoensperger at the imperial city of Augsburg, on Saint Bonifacius day, in the year 1486]. In the foreground the figures of five men are outlined. These no doubt are intended to represent the masters in medicine, since the following names are inscribed below these outlines in the original:

Galenus, Avicenna, Plinius, Serapion and Dioscorides. Back of
these figures stands a prescription counter, on which can be seen
a book, scale, mortar, and a number of boxes. At the table the

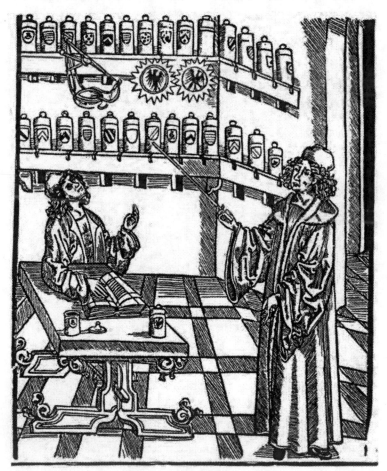

Fig. 13.
(From a book of 1505).

ancient prototype of the apprentice is lustily pounding away at
some obdurate root or herb, whilst the spirits of the great fathers
of medicine stand before his mind as worthy sires for emulation
and hallowed veneration.

Figure 13 is taken from a work by Hieronymus Brunschwygk, entitled "Das nüv Buch der rechten kunst zu distilliren. Ouch von Marsilio Ficino vn andrer hochberömpter Artzte natürliche vnd gute kunst zu behalten den gesunden leib vnd zu vertryben die kranckheit mit erlengerung des lebens," [The new book on the art of distilling. Also the natural and good art of preserving a healthy body, to banish disease and to prolong life; by Marsilio Ficino and other renowned doctors. Published in 1505]. An earlier edition of this work was published by Grueninger at Strassburg in 1500.

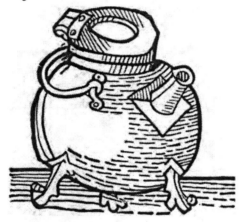

Fig. 14.

A WATER JUG.

In these illustrations of Middle Age pharmacies, it is to be noted that, in place of labels, the containers bear the coats of arms of titled families and the badges of cities.

The attaching of coats of arms to furniture and all household utensils was much practiced in those days, and as in all probability special containers were not made for pharmacies thus early, such bottles and jars were chosen as could be found in the market, so that although these escutcheons, etc., could serve no useful purpose, they certainly proved to be quite ornamental.

Whether or not a system of numbering was in use for determining the contents, as in later centuries, is not known. The stars in Figure 13 probably served for ornamental purposes only.

In the "Ortus sanitatis," the containers in which medicinal substances were preserved, find frequent illustration.   Distilled water

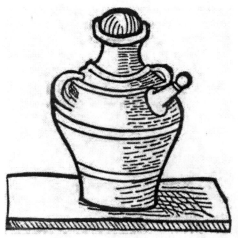

Fig. 15.
A VINEGAR JUG.

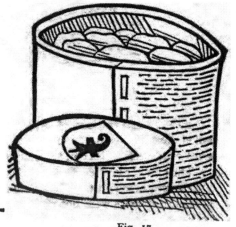

Fig. 16.
WOODEN BOX.

Fig. 17.
WOODEN BOX.

and vinegar were kept in earthen jars, Figures 14 and 15.   Small quantities of dry substances were kept in small wooden boxes, Figure 16.   Roots and herbs in larger quantities were kept in

large, round wooden boxes, like Figure 17. Figure 18, taken
from the same work, depicts a peddler offering "red earth"
for sale. Red earth was used for a variety of purposes; as
a polishing powder, as a paint, as a background in the process of gilding, and by others as a curative agent. In the text

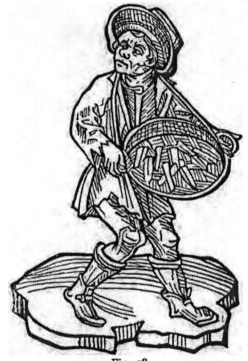

Fig. 18.
ANCIENT PEDDLER.

it is described as a "Bolus armenus vel lutum armenum," and
Armenia is specially emphasized as its source of introduction.
   The laboratory of the Middle Age pharmacist appears in
Figure 19. An apprentice is handling a tripod over an open
fire under the direction of his master, but the furniture of a
laboratory of the Middle Ages was by no means so limited as
would appear from the illustration. The medical works of those
days speak of the multiplicity of apparatus and utensils then in
use.

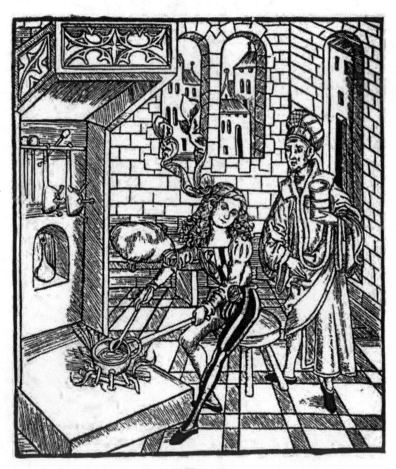

Fig. 19.

PHARMACAL LABORATORY, A. D. 1500.

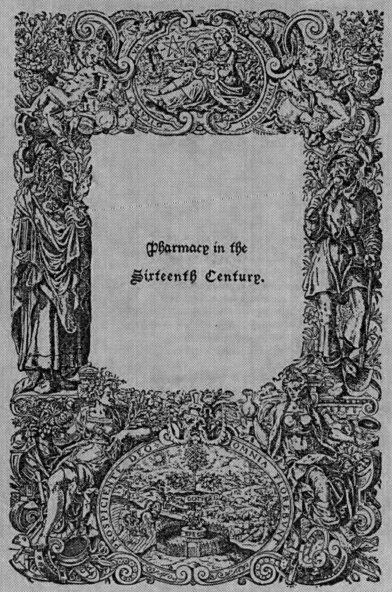

Pharmacy in the Sixteenth Century.

Fig. 20.
(From "Book of Herbs," 1586).

(33)

In my shop of drugs are stored
Many things of sweet accord,
Spices with sugar I combine,
Enemas and purges I divine.
To strengthen the weak and the sickly,
Refreshing draughts I furnish quickly.
All these, with utmost care,
On prescriptions I prepare.

HANS SACHS,
"True Description of all Professions." 1568.

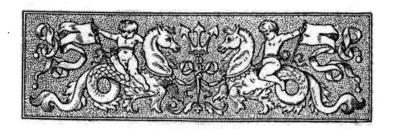

Chapter Three.

Pharmacy in the Sixteenth Century.

GURE 21, from the "Reformation of Pharmacy, An Illustrated Book of Herbs;" by Otto Brunfels, of Mayence, depicts the interior of a sixteenth century drug-store. The "Reformation of Pharmacy" was originally an essay presented by Dr. Brunfels, then city physician of Berne, to the Honorable Council of that city. At the instance of his widow, the work was published at

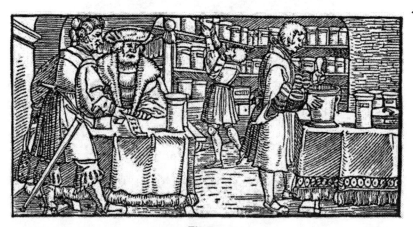

Fig. 21.
DRUG-STORE, A. D. 1536.

Strasburg ten years later, with this picture on its title page. From this illustration it is obvious that labels were beginning to take the place of the coats-of-arms of the earlier pharmacy. Brunfels describes with great care the containers for each kind of medicine. Dry, delicate and aromatic herbs should be so preserved as to prevent stagnation or a too ready escape of the odoriferous principles with which their medicinal virtues are intimately associated. Moist drugs must be kept in silver, glass or horn jars. Eye unguents must be preserved in china, whereas marrow, lard and crude matter of like character may be kept in zinc boxes. Oils are best kept in glass. Species aromatic in gold or silver material. Theriac, if genuine, would be worthy of a golden box, but one of zinc or lead will answer.

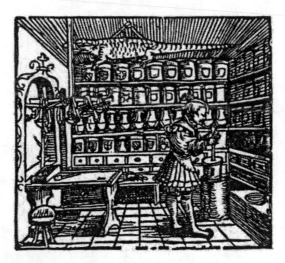

Fig. 22.

DRUG-STORE, A. D. 1548.

The elaborate table coverings in Fig. 21, indicate that some care was taken to please the eye. By way of ornamentation, to attract the customer and to give the store a more fantastic appearance, it was decorated with strange animal forms, plants and other curiosities. Fig. 22 (from "A Book of Confections, and a Family Physician," by G. Ryff, of Strassburg, 1548), shows a stuffed crocodile for this purpose. This picture vividly recalls the description of an apothecary given by Shakespere fifty years later in "Romeo and Juliet:"

I do remember an apothecary,—
And hereabouts he dwells,—which late I noted
In tatter'd weeds, with overwhelming brows
Culling of simples ; meagre were his looks,
Sharp misery had worn him to the bones :
And in his needy shop a tortoise hung,
An alligator stuffed, and other skins
Of ill-shaped fishes ; and about his shelves
A beggarly account of empty boxes,
Green earthen pots, bladders and musty seeds,
Remnants of packthread and old cakes of roses,
Were thinly scattered to make up a show.

"A True Description of all Professions," published at Frankfurt in 1568, with wood-cuts by Jost Amman, and words by the

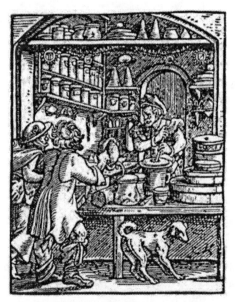

Fig. 23.
DRUG-STORE, 1568.

poetic son of St. Crispin, Hans Sachs, devotes a cut to the
apothecaries guild (Figure 23). Above the shelves proper are
cones of sugar. Ryff ("Family Physician") says : "Honey and
sugar are the druggist's chief stock in trade. He uses it for his
confects, electuaries, preserves, syrups, julips and other precious

mixtures." Sugar, moreover, was one of the main sources of income for the sixteenth century druggist. This century was peculiarly unkind to the apothecaries, especially as they were involved in perpetual contentions with the physicians.

From the twelfth century until the Reformation, Arabian pharmacy, with its complicated mixtures, had been in the ascendancy. But with the period of the Renaissance and the discovery of printing, came the study of the Greek classics, and Arabianism, with its complex therapeutics was banished from occidental medicine. The teachings of Hippocrates and other Greeks, and Averroes, dwelt largely on the dietetic treatment of the sick. The services of the apothecary were, therefore, less demanded than formerly.

The position of the pharmacist in England was a relatively high one. The separation of pharmacal from medical practice was almost complete in the sixteenth century in England. Bulleyn, " Queen Anne Bulleyn's cousin," a prominent apothecary, laid down the following rules for the practice of pharmacy :

> The apothecary must first serve God ; foresee the end, be cleanly, and pity the poor. His place of dwelling and shop must be cleanly, to please the senses withal. His garden must be at hand with plenty of herbs, seeds and roots. He must read Dioscorides. He must have his mortars, stills, pots, filters, glasses, boxes, clean and sweet. He must have two places in his shop, one most clean for physic and the base place for chirurgic stuff. He is neither to decrease nor diminish the physician's prescription. He is neither to buy nor sell rotten drugs. He must be able to open well a vein, for to help pleurisy. He is to meddle only in his own vocation, and to remember that his office is only to be the physician's cook.

These rules, save, perhaps the last, are not so antiquated as to merit oblivion. Long after the division of the practice of medicine the apothecaries continued subordinate to the medical practitioner, who used all possible endeavors to subject them to his will. Jealousies arose between the two classes which occasioned endless disputes.

In France these disputes assumed a somewhat farcical phase. The physicians, enraged at advice being given by apothecaries, determined to starve them out, and by prescribing only simple remedies from herbalists they subdued the rebel apothecary, obliging him to take the following oath :

> I swear and promise before God, the Author and Creator of all things, One in Spirit and divided in Three Persons, eternally blessed, that I will observe strictly the following articles :

First.   I promise to live and die in the Christian faith.

Second.   To love and honor my parents to the utmost; also, to honor, respect and render service, not only to the medical doctors who have imparted to me the precepts of pharmacy, but also to my teachers and masters from whom I have learned my trade.

Third.   Not to slander any of my ancient teachers or masters, whoever they may be ; also, to do all I can for the honor, glory and majesty of physic.

Fourth.   Never to teach to ungrateful persons or fools the secrets and mysteries of the trade ; never to do anything rashly without the advice of a physician, or from the sole desire of gain ; never to give any medicine or purge to invalids afflicted with acute disease without first consulting one of the faculty.

Fifth.   Never to examine woman privately, unless by great necessity, or to apply to them some necessary remedy; never to divulge the secrets confided to me.

Sixth.   Never to administer poisons, nor recommend their administration, even to our greatest enemies, nor to give drinks to produce abortion, without the advice of a physician, also to execute accurately their prescriptions, without adding or diminishing anything contained in them, that they may in every respect be prepared "*secundem artem.*"

Seventh.   Never to use any succedaneum or substitute without the advice of others wiser than myself; to disown and shun as a pestilence the scandalous and pernicious practices of quacks, empirics and alchymists, which exist to the great shame of the magistrates who tolerate them.

Lastly.   To give aid and assistance indiscriminately to all who employ me, and to keep no stale or bad drug in my shop.   May God continue to bless me so long as I continue to obey these things.

In Belgium, where the profession had become overcrowded, it became necessary to limit the number.   An act was passed in 1582 that no one should open an apothecary shop who had not previously studied pharmacy during three years, and adduced theoretical and practical demonstrations of his knowledge and capabilities, and taken the oath of the body corporate.   In 1585 a further act was enacted regarding the sale of arsenic.   In Bruges, in 1683, on complaint of the apothecaries, medical practitioners were forbidden to dispense under heavy penalty.   During the first three days only of the annual fair were charlatans and tooth-drawers allowed in the town.   Over-crowding had left its imprint on the profession elsewhere, notably in Amsterdam, Basel, Venice, Nuremburg, etc., with the result that the devices for making money that the apothecaries were compelled to adopt, threatened general disorganization.   To mitigate this evil, the Emperor Charles V, at the Congress of Augsburg in 1548, decreed as follows :

" It having come to our ears that deteriorated and spurious drugs are being dispensed on physicians' prescriptions, which, if taken into the system, will do more harm than good, we do herewith decree, that it is our will that the authorities in matters pertaining to the apothecaries' trade, should annually visit and inspect their shops, and also fix the values of all materials there found, so that the buyer shall in no way be deceived." *

This decree appears to have been heeded by the authorities and to have borne fruit, for on July 8, 1551, the council of Nuremburg passed a number of resolutions, one of which ordains that "in future no new drug-store shall be established, nor shall a new one take the place of any which may be discontinued." When in 1578 Valerius Pfister found his business declining, the city council ordered the other sixth druggist to buy his shop, promising the latter that no new pharmacy "except the hospital pharmacy" (which was the eighth), should be tolerated in Nuremburg.

Individual cities had instituted inspection of pharmacies at an earlier day, Bruges in 1497 and Nuremburg in 1442. But in the latter city all drug-stores were visited in one day; hence the inspection cannot have been very thorough. Since pharmacists, even at this early day, were accused of overcharging, the evil was regulated by affixing a specific selling price to each drug. Though the purchasing power of coin at that time is no certain measure of its value now, yet the following apothecary's bill of the sixteenth century may throw some light on the prices of drugs:

SIR PAULUS BECHAIM.

March 29th.	Two draughts......................	64 *pfg.*
30th.	One heart-water....................	42
	Fresh cassia.......................	56
	Rose honey........................	16
	Spices and herbs..................	56
31st.	Spices and herbs..................	42
	Minth	4
April 30th.	One heart-water....................	42
	Manna........................ 4 *lb.*	18
	Head-wash........................	18
	Heart-flower	6
	Electuary.........................	38
	Liver-water.......................	24
	Draught..........................	26

Summa   2 *fl.* 2 *lb.*   8 *pfg.*

Paid, April 30th, 1551.

ALBRECHT PFISTER.

* From "Collegium Pharmaceuticum" of the city of Nuremburg, p. 149.

Pharmacist Albrecht Pfister, who receipted this bill, was born in 1500 and died in 1564. He owned a drug-store in Binder Street, Nuremburg, still in existence and known as the " Star-Pharmacy."

The condition of the drug trade is very lucidly pictured in a memorial of the druggists of Nuremburg, in 1581, to the council, defending themselves against ·charges made by physicians. Many complaints therein enumerated are even now frequently heard ; a few extracts from this memorial will therefore be of interest :

May it please the Honorable Council to lend ear to our complaints, and in conformity therewith to see fit, in such a manner, to protect our interests, that henceforth we shall not be unduly oppressed by the physicians, and that each of us shall be enabled to enjoy the just results of his labors. The following, honorable sirs, forms the substance of our complaint :

1. The sale of all confections, formerly dispensed by us, has now fallen into the hands of the sugar dealer.

2. Counter sales are now made by all the large spice and cheap corner grocery shops, thus robbing the druggist of a source of profit that he is justly entitled to.

3. The sale of sundries, such as sealing wax, fumigating pastiles, paper ink and pens, is now taking place in common huckster shops.

4. The sugar dealers are not only selling confections but also all kinds of fruit juices, electuaries of quinces, and all such preserves that do not deterio· rate in the course of a year.

5. All distilled waters, oils, and the like, which were formerly kept by druggists only, are now indiscriminately sold by any ignoramus who imagines himself qualified to engage in this traffic.

6. Unguenta and Emplastra, which certainly belong to the exclusive field of pharmacy, are now dispensed by barbers and ignorant physicians, who are neither justified by precedent nor by qualification to handle these things.

7. Now, many expensive *medicamenta* are, every year, carried over and deteriorate, because the doctors do not prescribe them, and they prove a total loss to the druggist. Of such medicines we will but enumerate the fruit juices, the purging elixir of roses, etc. ; furthermore, the "*electuaria solutiva, tam in liquida, quam in solida forma*," and the "*massa pillularum et trochiscorum genera.*"

In this summary it will be noticed the delightful *confectiones* are entirely forgotten. *Species* and *confectiones comfortativae* are also overlookēd. The principal cause of this state of things is, that the " physicians are eternally devising new and extraordinary remedies." After dilating upon other more or less impor· tant points, the memorial further says :

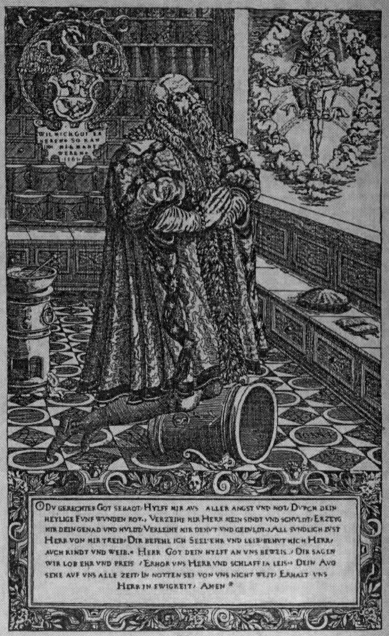

Fig. 24.

AN APOTHECARY, 1565.

* Translation—Foot-note, page 43.

"We were pained to learn that the physicians have charged us with selling adulterated and injurious drugs, and declare that the public had on this account withdrawn its patronage from us. Self-preservation and honor demand that we no longer remain quiet under these accusations. Albeit, there may be persons who do not wish to deal with us, there are, nevertheless, numbers that prefer to be treated by us, and if we deny them the succor asked for, and send them to the physician, they will be displeased and go without any treatment whatever. This much, also, is certain, that if we would dispense medicines in all cases where we are called upon to prescribe, we would shortly have more patients than the physicians. We have, furthermore, abundant proof that the physicians frequently overstep the boundary line of *their* field. They, for instance, prescribe in German, so that any barber or old woman can prepare the medicine, and the druggist is ignored."

No further proof is needed that the golden age of pharmacy is not to be found in the past.

Figure 24, from an etching dated 1565, in the Germanic Museum, depicts a representative sixteenth century pharmacist, named Cyriacus Schnaus, kneeling on his mortar absorbed in offering a fervent prayer. Schnaus practiced the black art, and is mentioned with the printers of his time. He is known to have been engaged in literary pursuits.

In Germany at the close of this century the services of the apothecary had become so important that in times of war regular field pharmacies were organized. Works were published in 1582 and 1596 giving directions for furnishing traveling and field pharmacies. The Nuremburg complaint made against the spicers and sugar-bakers indicates that grocers and herbalists were becoming separate occupations, and that the pharmacist was assuming more the position of a professional man and less that of a tradesman, considerably to his pecuniary detriment. Toward the end of the present century this tendency to separation became especially marked in the Grocer's Company of England, which then included the apothecaries. The "Stationarii" and "Confectionarii" of the thirteenth century had become merged in the fourteenth, but were now beginning a final separation into grocers, spicers, sugar-bakers, and apothecaries.

* O Thou most righteous God, by Thine five holy wounds, stand by me in my anguish and want. Forgive me my sins and my shortcomings. Show me Thy mercy and tenderness, and fortify me with patience and humbleness of heart. Deliver me from all sinful lust. In Thy hands I place body and soul. Protect me, O Lord, also my child and wife. O God, prove unto us Thy power. Thee we honor and praise. Listen to us, O Lord, and sleep lightly. Let Thine eye rest upon us at all times. Be not far from us in our suffering. Keep us, O Lord, in all eternity. Amen.

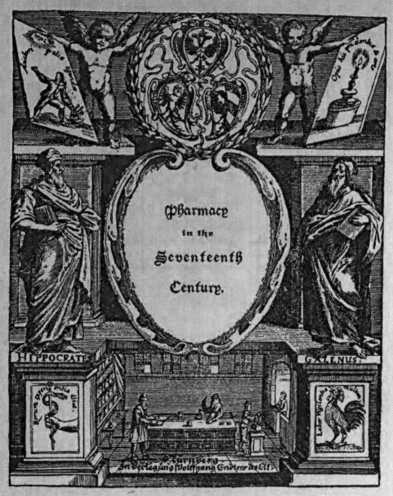

Fig. 25.

(From a " Medical Code," 1652).

" What once we did as Nature's secret rate,
We now do coolly investigate,
And what once Dame Nature organized,
That is by us now crystallized."

—FAUST.

40

Chapter Four.

Pharmacy in the Seventeenth Century.

OD-ENGRAVING, which had attained its highest development during the sixteenth century, was, at the beginning of the seventeenth century, supplanted by copper-plate, which had been gradually growing in favor. The wood-cut, from the time of the Thirty-years War down to the nineteenth century. fell into almost entire disuse. To the Englishman, Thomas Bewick, is due what might properly be called the rediscovery of the woodcut, early in the present century. Owing to the greater expense of the copper-print, the seventeenth century books contain much fewer illustrations than those of the time immediately precedent. This dearth of illustrations is discernible in the pharmacal publications of the period under consideration.

Fig. 25 is a copperprint from the title-page of an ordinance concerning the tax regulations of drugs in the city of Nuremburg in 1652. It depicts the ancient classical medical authorities. To the left is the Greek physician, Hippocrates, and to the right Galenus of Pergamus, who practiced in Rome.

The numerous additions to the materia medica of the seventeenth century brought about a considerable change in the equipment of pharmacies. Two causes were influential in bringing about this increase in the materia medica,— the extensive introduction of American drugs, and the adoption of chemical remedies. The latter had, in isolated instances, been employed in the sixteenth century. The introduction of chemical remedies into therapeutics is largely due to "Philippus Theophrastus Bombastus, of Hohenheim," known as "Paracelsus" (Figure 26).

He was born in 1490 near Einsiedeln, in the Canton Schwyz, and began his medical studies in the University of Basel. His extensive knowledge of the natural sciences, acquired during his sojourn at other renowned universities, his close observations during his extensive travels over Europe, together with his

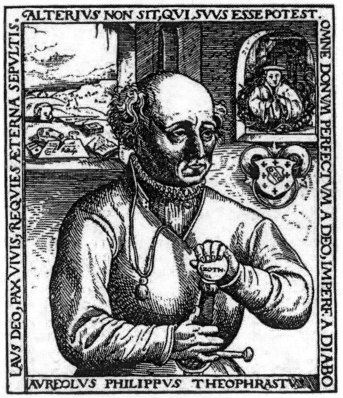

Fig. 26.

PARACELSUS.

(From a work, 1568).

knowledge of medicine, eminently qualified him for the duties of city physician of Basel, which office he accepted in 1526. The following year he lectured at the university.

In imitation of Luther, who had inaugurated his church reformation by burning the bulls of the Pope, Paracelsus began his reformatory activity by burning the highly prized works of the Arabian, *Avicenna,* "the Prince of Physicians," and those of other medical authorities, on St. John's day, in the year 1527, exclaiming, "I have burned all these books so that all misery may be carried away with their smoke." Like Luther, he discarded Latin, and wrote the greater number of his books in German, the language of the people, a proceeding directly opposed to all customs and usages. He afterward boasted that he had not read a book in ten years. He protested that his shoebuckles were more learned than Galen and Avicenna. He had a dogma of his own. This man, in whom learning and quackery were so singularly combined, "believed that the human body was a microcosm," which corresponded to the "macrocosm," and contained in itself all parts of visible nature, sun, moon, stars and the poles of heaven. Disease, according to his mystical conception, was not natural but spiritual. Therefore some remedy had to be introduced which was antagonistic, not to the disease in a physical sense, but to the spiritual seed of the disease. These remedies were called "Arcana," a word which implied a mysterious connection between the remedy and the *essence* of the disease and in its relation to medicine, somewhat akin to the word "specific," at the present day.

Great importance was attached to chemically prepared remedies, as containing the essence or spiritual quality of the material from which they were derived. His followers were therefore known as "chemical" physicians. The most notorious of that school in England was a certain Anthony. Paracelsus still accepted the old physical elements, but attributed qualities to them more in conformity with modern views. Altogether he held that his "arcana" were semi-spiritual beings like the "quinta essentia" of Aristotle ; he nevertheless believed that he could dissolve or extract them by means of water, alcohol, or acids. While his principle was fallacious and led to many errors, it nevertheless contributed to the displacement of the complicated galenical preparations by the discovery of tinctures, extracts, and metallic salts, thereby very materially simplifying the art of prescribing. He believed God had ordained that man should be guided by the outward forms and psychical impressions of objects in nature, in applying remedies in disease; and he accordingly chose his remedies, not on the principle of their action, but on their resemblance or sympathetic relations to the patient and his disease.   In this wise the notorious teachings of the "Signatures" were revived, which under different names had swayed the minds of men in ancient times.

On the strength of these and similar earlier notions the doctrines of "similia similibus curantur" were at a later day adopted

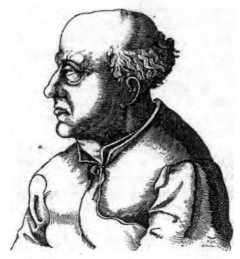

Fig. 27.

PARACELSUS, BOMBAST VON HOHENHEIM.

(From a wood-cut of 1565).

by Hahnemann, as a fundamental principle in homœopathy. After the death of Paracelsus his adherents rapidly multiplied.

At the beginning of the seventeenth century two antagonistic parties lay claim to the true science of medicine,—the Galenists and the Paracelsists.   Their animosity grew deeper and deeper, and whilst the Thirty-years War was devastating Germany, battle-cries of a different character were influencing the minds of contending parties in the realm of Æsculapius.   But the Galenico-Arabian school, which had succeeded in 1643 at Paris in having an edict issued forbidding the use of metallic salts, was finally vanquished.   The medicinal preparations of Paracelsus (tinctures, extracts, and chemicals) secured recognition in pharmacy.

Chemistry, which thus far had been subordinated to alchemistic hypotheses, triumphantly entered the laboratories of the seventeenth century, and electuaries like mithridates and theriac were supplanted by more strictly scientific preparations. The picturesquely descriptive methods of the old alchemists were not suited to the more simple and scientific manipulations instituted. When chemistry, therefore, entered the service of medicine, more rational

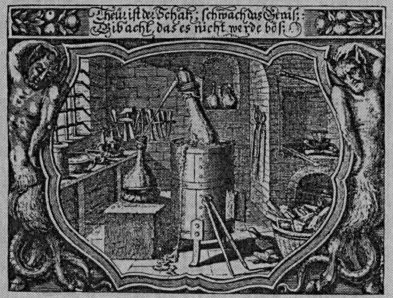

Fig. 28.
PHARMACAL LABORATORY, 1663.

modes of expression were adopted. One Oswald Troll, physician to the Prince of Anhalt, made himself conspicuous in 1608 by publishing his "Basilica chymica," in which he gives very intelligible directions for the preparation of chemicals. The Parisian druggist, Nicholas Lemery, was particularly instrumental in paving the way for this innovation, by publishing his work, "Cours de Chimie," in 1675. This work evinced a lucid style unknown before his day, which soon secured for it a translation into English, German, Spanish, Italian, and Latin.

The principal changes connected with pharmacy in the seventeenth century, took place in the laboratory. Some of these are to be observed in Figure 28, taken from a religious work of 1663. On the portable stove is a distilling apparatus, now out of use, which consists of a simple glass retort and helm or cover, known as an "alembic," from "αμβιξ (*a cover*)." Possibly, at this very moment, the liquor crani humani was in process of distillation, for just about this time the notion prevailed that all medicines for man must be obtained out of the microcosmos itself. Nicolas Lemery says, in "Cours de Chimie," that the officinal human skull, "cranium humanum," must be procured from a young, vigorous, and but recently killed and as yet unburied man, to secure all the "principia activa." This distillate was good for the "falling sickness," gout, apoplexy, somnolency, and dysmenorrhœa. It was a diaphoretic and a powerful antidote for poisons. From this it would appear that the old fetichism held its own in the realm of therapeutics. In 1663 the chemist Joseph Bechler, in his "Parnassus Medicinalis Illustratus," enumerates the following diseases that the different parts of the human body will cure, as follows :

Powdered human bone in red wine will cure dysentery. The marrow and oil distilled from bone is good for rheumatism. Prepared human skull is a sure cure for the falling sickness. Moss grown on a skull is an hæmostatic. Mummy dissolves coagulated blood, relieves cough and pain in the spleen, and is also very beneficial in flatulency and delayed menstruation. Human fat, when properly rubbed into the skin, restores weak limbs. The wearing of a belt made of human skin facilitates labor and mitigates its pain. Water distilled from human hair and mixed with honey promotes the growth of hair," etc.

Fig. 29 (from the same work as the preceding picture) shows the interior of an apothecary's shop. It does not present any striking improvement over those of the previous century, though the apothecaries had advanced in scientific attainments to a marked degree. They not only cultivated chemistry, but also earnestly entered upon the study of botany. From the total lack of system in botanical works of the day, it was extremely difficult to recognize plants by their mere description. Cæsalpinus, professor of botany at Pisa, had, at the close of the sixteenth century, endeavored to classify the plant world in fifteen classes, according to their flowers and fruits, but his work was not generally accepted, and the necessity of illustrations to convey correct ideas of plants, was much greater than at the present day.

The botanical works of the sixteenth century were therefore elaborately supplied with wood-cuts. In the seventeenth century, the copper-print takes their place. The first large work of the kind illustrated with the latter, is the "Hortus Eystettensis," published by the druggist, Basilius Besler, in 1613. The illustra-

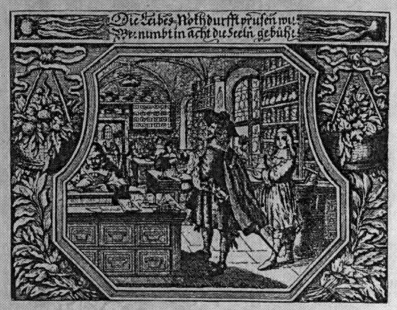

Fig. 29.
DRUG-STORE, 1663.

tions are very artistic and true to nature, and hardly eclipsed by modern productions. The plants are classified without reference either to their structure or time of florescence. The author could not, however, abstain from incorporating his portrait, of which Fig. 30 is a reduced copy. The margin bears this inscription :

"Basil. Besler Noricus, artis pharmaceuticæ, chymicæ amator singularis rei herbariæ studiosus aetatis suae 51 anno 1612."

This would indicate that he was born in 1561. From the annals of the Collegii Pharmaceutici it appears that he was the proprie-

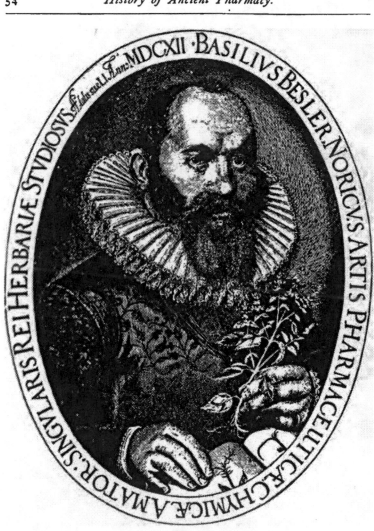

Fig. 30.

A PHARMACIST OF 1613.

tor of the Haymarket pharmacy in Nuremburg from 1586 to 1629, when he died. This drug-store was discontinued in 1792. After the death of Besler, botany was extensively studied by the druggists of Nuremburg. To this end, they in 1668 associated themselves with the physicians, and thereafter it was their custom to make botanical excursions in common, in the fall and and spring of the year, and such plants which were found to possess peculiar medicinal properties, were classified and described in the Annals of the College of Physicians. A trip of this kind was called an " herbation." These herbations ordinarily wound up with a banquet in a neighboring town, or in a club-room in the city. These gatherings were anything but dry and formal affairs, as the surviving specimens of their poetry revel in melodious rhyme.

That excessive abstinence did not injure the physician and pharmacist becomes evident from the magnitude of the accompanying bill from among the archives of the Nuremburg "Collegii Pharmaceutici"

To Mr. WURFFBAIN'S HERBATION, *May 16, 1698, at which nineteen persons were present.*

2 Dishes Stew.............................Florin,	3.20
2 Meat pies, 12 chickens and veal.................. "	7.40
2 Dishes, 3 sour tongues.......................... "	1.48
1 Dish, 8 lbs. fish .... "	2.40
1 " 6 Geese .... "	3 36
2 Dishes, 12 chickens .... "	4.48
1 Dish, 2 Rabbits and 10 wild ducks............... "	4 14
2 Dishes, 36 cheese cakes......................... "	1 12
2 " Lobsters............................. "	1.44
2 " Hop balls .... "	1.36
1 Westphalian ham.............................. "	2.00
Collation .... "	3.00
Wheat and rye bread .... "	.46
1 Barrel of Wine and 1 pail .... "	24.48
Waiter .... "	.45
2 Dishes of asparagus............................ "	1.44
6 Plates of raddish.............................. "	.24

Florin, 62.45
CHRISTOPH ZINNERER,
Wine Merchant.

N. B.—Together, 19 persons. Makes for each person, 4 Florin and 4 Kreuzer.

These gentlemen evidently knew how to combine business with pleasure. In any event it is apparent that the druggists of Nuremberg, at least, did not maintain an indifferent attitude

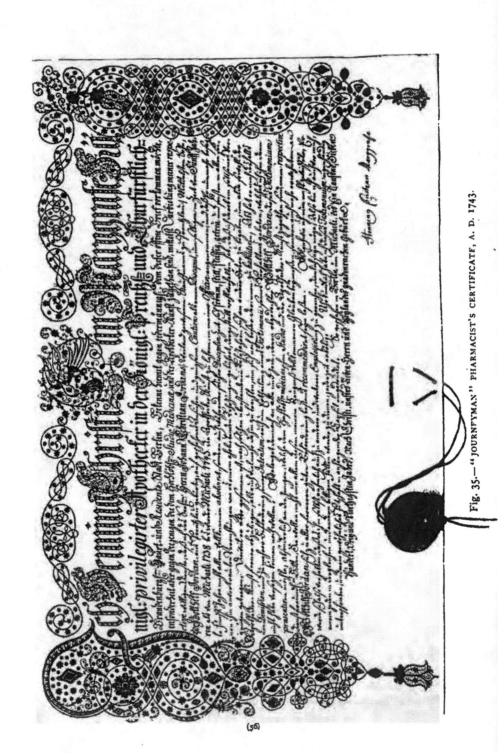

Fig. 35.—"JOURNEYMAN" PHARMACIST'S CERTIFICATE, A. D. 1743.

toward the natural sciences, and that they contributed a very respectable share to the fundamental material upon which, in the eighteenth century, Becher, Stahl, Lavoisier, Linnæus, Cadwallader Colden, Steele, Priestley and others reared the grand superstructures of chemistry and botany.

The education of the pharmacist was still largely based on his trade experiences, although those who adopted the profession were obliged to possess some knowledge of Latin. The apprenticeship lasted from five to six years, and at the end of this time the apprentice was, by his master, created a "journeyman." The certificate issued on such occasions was of great elegance, frequently elaborately ornamented, and written on parchment. The accompanying illustration is a reduced copy of one of those issued in 1743, the original of which exists in the Germanic Museum.

The journeyman apothecary was usually obliged to pass an examination before the Decanum Collegii at the time of applying for a situation. The duties of a drug clerk were embodied in the following regulations :

Every journeyman apothecary shall take an oath that he will faithfully serve, not only his master, but also the members of the community at large. That he will prepare all medicines "secundem artem," and of pure drugs, whether they be such as are annually examined by the authorities or not. That he will dispense no poison, opiate or emmenagogue without the knowledge of the master, or endanger the life of any one by his carelessness. That he will not deliberately change a physician's prescription, and will abstain from excessive indulgence in intoxicating drinks, and will at all times set a good example to the apprentice. That he will not leave the shop without the knowledge of the master, and particularly not absent himself at night. That he will be devoted to his master, to the Visitatori Medico, and to each of the doctors of the incorporated Collegio Medico. He shall swear that he will do all this according to his best ability."

On assuming control of a pharmacy as a proprietor, he was required to pass a supplementary examination. Apothecaries ranked with the third estate. When, in the seventeenth century, it became customary for apothecaries in Germany to take an academic course, they claimed to rank with the learned class, and emphasized this by wearing "caput-coats" and sabres. Tradespeople were not allowed to wear sabres, hence the police interfered and suppressed this demonstration of their budding greatness. Thereupon the combined apothecaries of Nuremburg petitioned the Council, dilating upon the injustice of the action taken against them. They refer to the fact that in other cities, Frankfurth, Ulm, Strassburg, Augsburg and Vienna, while trades-people were debarred from the wearing of sabres, apothecaries, nevertheless, are allowed to do so. This is no more than just, since many have matriculated at universities, some have attended academies, and others have even graduated as doctors. " This injunction," they further say, " rests all the more heavily upon us, when we consider that our profession is not a trade. but is in reality a free art."

This petition, whose results are not recorded, clearly demonstrates that the social position of the pharmacists then, as now, was somewhat disputed in Germany, when contrasted with that of the technical practitioners, the learned and the tradesmen. That the prominent position of the pharmacist should have led satirists to attack their short-comings was but natural. Father " Abraham a Sancta Clara," in " Description of All Professions and Trades," published in 1699, usually deals very leniently with them, but can not abstain from a gentle reprimand. " On the whole," he says, " the druggists can not be too highly praised, and, if it were possible, their glory should be written in lines of potable gold which they know how to prepare so skillfully. Their daily life also is, for the most part, religious and faultless. Still one also finds some who have many 'scruples' in their shops, but never allow 'scruples' to interfere in their dealings with their fellow man. They boast of having in stock all kinds of Medicamenta, such as Emollientia, Resolventia, Condensentia, Aperientia, Constipantia, Attrahentia, Repercutientia, Abstergentia, Expurgantia, Attenuantia, Illinentia, Maturantia, Conglutinantia, Cientia, Expellentia, etc., but more frequently one finds there Fallentia ; that is, superannuated species, that are more harmful than beneficial to the patient. This results from a habit they have of buying, at a cheap price, goods that have been kept in stock at some grocers from time immemorial, and that smell worse than Lazarus in his grave. Then you will frequently meet with a druggist who has spent his entire apprenticeship behind the mortar, and knows nothing about any 'crout' (herb) excepting it be the 'sour' kind, which he will recognize when it is cooked with a saddle of pork. Then, again, he will make more mistakes than the children of the prophet in the days of Elisha, who gathered in the bitter colocynth in place of healing herbs."

Moscherosch, a seventeenth century satirist, displays a cynically sarcastic feeling toward the medical world. In a book published in 1643, he says:

"The drug-shops are veritable arsenals, and the keepers thereof, the druggists, are gunsmiths in the service of the Medicis." "For," says he, "everything you find in their shops remind one of war and war-implements. There is, in the first place, the *mortar*, with its very appropriate name, which seems to barricade and break down the gates of the human system. The syringe, when it projects the enema, may be likened unto a pistol. The pills are the musket balls. The Medici stand for grim death himself. The Medicamentia purgantia are the genuine fire of purgatorium ; the barbers are the devils, and the drug shop is a diminutive hades, whilst the patient represents the poor, lost and condemned soul. The druggists display in their shops slips of paper covered with strange and wonderful hieroglyphs, that neither Vitzliputzli or Tlaloc of Mexico, nor Vlastu of Cusco, nor Quetzaalcoale of Chalula, nor the Chiappa Cariba, nor Tamaraca of Brazil, nor the Deumus of Calechut, nor the Novientium of the Alsacians of old, nor Mercurius of Speyer, nor the Natagia of the Tartars could decipher. The directions on these papers are usually preceded by ' Rec,' which in fact stands for per decem, and means that one prescription out of ten may help, or, more properly speaking, that of ten patients one *may* escape. They are called patients when they get into the hands of the fraternity, for from that moment they are condemned to suffer all the tortures of the damned."

" Furthermore, we meet with the word ' Ana,' which little word we derive from the French ' Asne ' or ' Ane ' (ass, fool), but really originates from Ana, the son of Zibeon, who invented the mule whilst herding his father's jackasses in the desert, and what word could more appropriately serve as an affix to a prescription than ' Ana,' since it takes but a careless ass to deprive an honest man of health and life. And then come the ' Drachmæ,' ' Unciæ,' ' Scrupuli,' ' Grana,' which have the shape of snakes, scorpions, and blind-worms, or at least are possessed of their

venom.   And all these beautiful things so comfort the patient
that his soul would almost take flight at sight of them.   And then
they apply such outlandish Indian and Turkish names to their
simples and other foul herbs, that one would imagine they
intended to conjure old Satan himself.   Such names for instance
as Opoponach, Tregoricarum, Petroselinum, Herba Borith,
Chamæspartion, Diaphæniconis, Scolopendrion, Diatrionpi-
pereon, Ophiostaphylon, Zoophthalmon, etc., which, upon close
examination, prove to be every-day parsley, cornflower, sanicle,
houseleek, tamarisk, juniper, red white, and yellow carrots, and
the like.   They call beans and lentils by such strange names to
tempt the patient's curiosity and induce him to pay an extra
price for the same.   Their mixtures are frequently so loathsome,
as to taste and odor, that one would expect to see the worst disease leave the body in haste to escape the contamination.   The
designation, *medical composita*, is another term to the point, for
when your druggist mixes pepper and mouse-dung, and runs it
through the mill, he may dispense it with a clear conscience, for
the patient is paying his money for a remedy that is clearly as
composite as the most exacting can desire."   That the druggists
should have haunted Moserosch in his dreams was not surprising.   One of these dreams he describes as follows :

"Then there followed a rabble of apothecaries with mortars,
jingling pestles, suppositoria, balneis mariæ, spatula, syringes, etc.,
which were all loaded with deadly missiles and powder.   They
also carried many boxes and bottles labeled 'medicine,' but in
reality containing poison only."

On another occasion he says : "After considering this matter
in all earnestness, I have come to the conclusion that all this
mourning and lamenting we are obliged to bestow upon the
dead, is really ushered in by the death-knell of the pestles on the
walls of the apothecaries' mortar, and only ceases with the
requiem and the sounding of the church bell."

It is of interest to note that in Italy, Zacchias, during this
century, advanced the view that there were self-generated poisons,
which is practically the view at present held concerning the
ptomaines and leucomaines of Selmi and Brieger.   In England
the existence of the Apothecaries Company seems to have placed
the social status of the apothecaries on a pretty well-defined

basis. The apothecary held in popular estimation and social dignity a place close to the physician. Physicians to the king were always accompanied by a staff of apothecaries. At the death-bed of Charles II both appear, and the administration of a volatile preparation from a human skull indicates that his disease was looked upon rather as "falling sickness" than apoplexy. The coffee-houses of this period, which were a leading

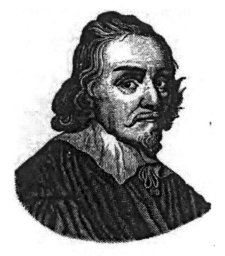

Fig. 36.
WILLIAM HARVEY.

feature of its social life, were visited by both physicians and apothecaries at certain times of the day under circumstances which show that both were regarded as members of a common profession.

William Harvey, the demonstrator of the circulation of the blood, was a staunch friend of the Apothecaries Company, and aided it with Charles I. He was a great student of pharmacology, and did not regard the use of animal products with much favor. He is often mentioned as visiting the coffee houses in company with apothecaries.

Pharmacy in English speaking America during the seventeenth century was largely based on English usages, more or less modified by practices derived from the Indians. As a result, a great many quack doctors and apothecaries sprang into prominence. These led Virginia to attempt the legal regulation of those who charged exorbitant fees, for in 1636 a law was passed regulating the fees of surgeons and apothecaries. Prominent among the early Virginian colonists who were at once surgeons and apothecaries was Dr. Edward Heldon, who had been a friend and pall-bearer of Shakespere. In Massachusetts, pharmacy was largely in the hands of the Indians, schoolmasters, old women and clergymen. The last were generally skilled apothecaries, who had learned pharmacy during periods of persecution, and practiced it for ostensible means of subsistence while preaching. The Rev. Jacob Green was at once lawyer, schoolmaster, miller, distiller, apothecary and physician. The witchcraft epidemic brought the practitioners of pharmacy into suspicion as selling poison for spells. As a rule the general merchants sold drugs to the apothecaries. As early as 1647 Giles Firmin, of Boston, had firmly established himself as devoting special attention to pharmacy. In 1646 the first store distinctly devoted to pharmacy was opened in Boston by William Davies.

Under the Duke of York's government, the province of New Jersey made an attempt to regulate the practice of apothecaries in 1664, which provided for penalties for injury. In New York there was a tendency exhibited to separate pharmacy from medicine. The quacks were exceedingly numerous in the city, and attempts were made to punish them for infraction of the Duke's laws passed in 1664. In 1689, when the revolution broke out, one work held in esteem in the practice of pharmacy, was Salmon's Herbal, originally printed in London in 1676. During the end of the seventeenth and early eighteenth century it was in high repute among American pharmacists.

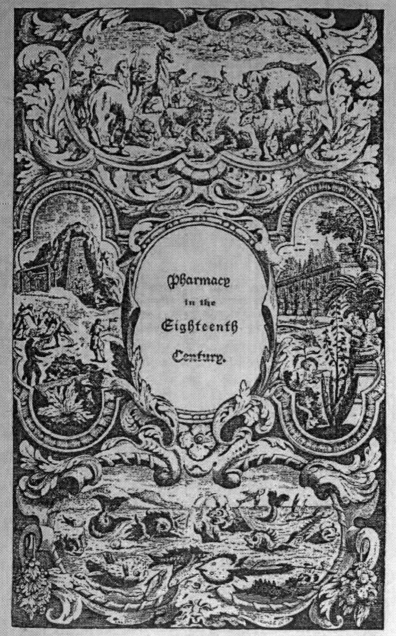

Fig. 37.
REPRESENTATION OF THE SOURCES OF THE MATERIA MEDICA.
(63)

" With glasses, boxes, round me stacked,
   And instruments together hurled,
Ancestral lumber, stuffed and packed—
   Such is my world ! and what a world ! "
                                    —FAUST.

Chapter Five.

Pharmacy in the Eighteenth Century.

E contentions of the Apothecaries and the Surgeons in England had resulted in the victory of apothecaries by the passage of Act 34, Henry VIII, in 1543, which protected them in counter prescribing. James I, in 1608, united them with the grocers, under the title of the "Warden and Commonalty of the Mystery of Grocers." To do this he revoked the charter of the old Grocers and Apothecaries Company. In 1617 the apothecaries were finally separated from the grocers, and the Apothecaries Company was created. This became a very important body, as the apothecary was now regarded as a practitioner of a medical specialty rather than a mere merchant. By degrees they gained so much public confidence, and began to take so active a part in the practice of medicine, that they had the audacity, when preparing an electuary or bolus, to reason on the propriety of its administration, to recommend a polypharmaceutical physician in preference to a prescriber of simples. To crown all, they began visiting patients themselves. This state of affairs occasioned a great variety of publications. The coarse wit and low abuse which abounded in these publications, are an evidence of the general ignorance of the contending parties, although some men of eminence might occasionally have been led into the errors of their contemporaries.

In 1665 a curious work was published by Dr. Record, "The Urinal of Physic." This contained an appendix, "A Treatise Concerning the Abuses of Physicians and Apothecaries." This treatise states that the latter "actually ventured to give purges,

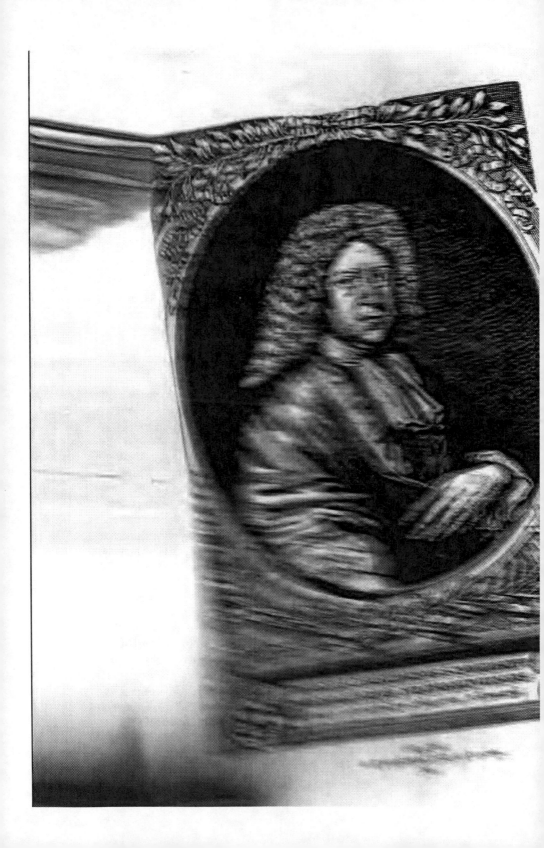

without the advice of the physician," which was in those days considered a serious offense. Every year added to the list of offenses. They were accused by the physicians of all sorts of misdeeds. In 1696 the College of Physicians established their own dispensary. The accusations continually directed against the apothecaries for selling bad medicines, furnished an excellent excuse for the formation of a joint-stock company; and the establishment of a laboratory at their hall for their own use, and for supplying members with drugs. This resulted in great injury to the manufacturing chemists and druggists; for, not content with supplying their own members, they obtained the orders of government for medical stores. The physicians, on the other hand, obtained the well known "Act for the Better Viewing of Drugs, etc., for Ten Miles Around London," which gave the apothecaries great offense, and occasioned the publication of a variety of squibs on both sides.

The pharmacists appear to have placed the profession on a sounder basis at this time preparatory to entering on a more promising era. That the apothecary's life had by this time experienced a vast improvement is shown by the more elaborate furnishing of the shops and laboratories.

Figure 37 on the title page depicted the provinces of nature that have at various times sustained the reign of Æsculapius. The picture is taken from the "Lexicon Pharmaceutico-Chymicum," by J. C. Sommerhoff, published in 1701. The marked preponderance of scroll-work at once stamps it as the product of a time when the renaissance style had degenerated into the pseudo-classical, and there were foreshadowings of the rococo period. Although the author, as pictured in Figure 38, wears a wig of very respectable proportions, he had not yet adopted the cue which became a craze in this pseudo-classical period, styled by the Germans "Die Zopfzeit" (the cue or tail period). But he lived to see King Frederic I introduce the cue into the army. The "Lexicon" was prefaced by poetic effusions by Sommerhoff's friend. The burden of these were the glorification of himself and his labors. Despite Sommerhoff's undeniable indebtedness to similar works of lesser scope, one of his friends indulges in the following:

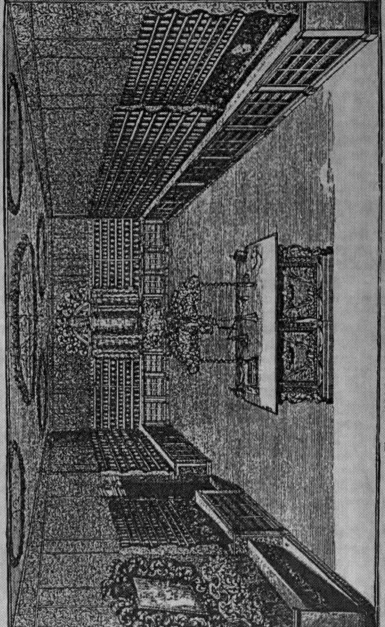

Fig. 30.—COURT PHARMACY AT RASTATT, A. D. 1700.

"May the result of his labors and pains in the past,
With his name, like pure gold, eternally last."

As a slight contribution to the realization of this wish, his portrait is here introduced, more especially as it serves at the same time to give an excellent idea of a representative pharmacist of the eighteenth century.

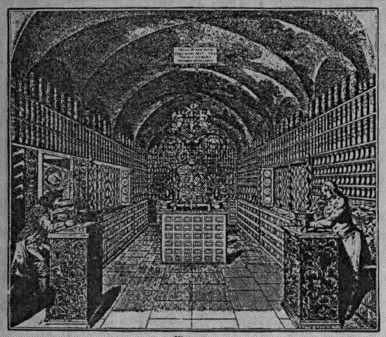

Fig. 40.

"STAR" PHARMACY AT NUREMBURG, A. D. 1710.

Fig. 39 depicts the court-pharmacy at Rastatt. A Latin inscription beneath the original reads: "This picture was dedicated to his most gracious master, the Commander-in-Chief of the army, Ludwig William, Count of Baden, by pharmacist Joh. L. Kellner." Kellner, who bought this pharmacy in 1697, had doubtless served under this count as a field-apothecary during his campaign against the Turks, since a field-pharmacy, preserved in this store for two hundred years, has recently been turned over to the Germanic Museum.

Fig. 40 represents the old "Star Pharmacy" at Nuremburg as it appeared before its removal to its present quarters in Binder street.　Much of the old furniture, boxes and bottles were brought over to the new stand at the time of the removal (1728), and remain to the present day.　The drawers are similar to

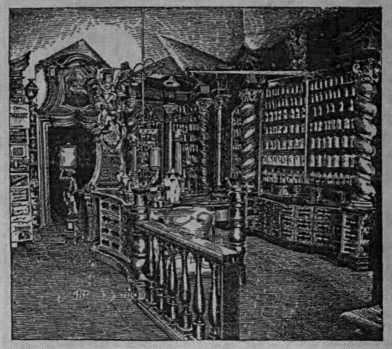

Fig. 41.
DRUG-STORE AT KLATTAU, A. D. 1733.

those of modern construction.　The bottles and containers for fluids, in lieu of ground stoppers, are furnished with a zinc cap, which is screwed down over the neck of the bottles.　The beautiful and richly-painted majolica ware, made in Italy and in use in Europe from the sixteenth century to the middle of the eighteenth, is to be seen in the "Star Pharmacy" at the present day.

When the ornamental majolica ware was supplanted by sober white china the pharmacies were deprived of much of their quaint and picturesque appearance.　The discovery of porcelain by Joh. F. Boettcher caused the more expensive majolica to fall into disuse. Boettcher began his chemical studies in a Berlin drug-store laboratory in 1701. His master, "Zorn," was engaged in alchemistic studies, and Boettcher had an excellent opportunity for learning the secrets of the art. His remarkably successful experiments soon gave him the reputation of being able, by the aid of some secret agency, to make gold. When this rumor reached the ears of King Frederic I of Prussia he ordered his arrest, but Boettcher, receiving timely warning, escaped to Saxony. Fearing that the fugitive would be kidnapped by the Prussians, who had demanded his extradition, he was brought to Dresden for greater safety. The Saxon ruler himself soon became convinced that Boettcher could make gold, and demanded the secret. Boettcher refused to comply, and was placed under strict surveillance, and practically imprisoned. He was coaxed by his guards to prosecute his experimental search for the philosopher's stone, and, in 1704, accidentally discovered brown jasper, and, in 1709, white porcelain. The latter, in 1710, became a staple manufacture of Meissen under the direction of Boettcher. From the middle of the eighteenth century it was in general use in the pharmacies.

Figure 41 shows the interior of a drug-store at Klattau, Bohemia. The present proprietor of the store relates that the pharmacy was established by the Jesuits in 1733, who controlled their own artisans, and introduced the same style of architecture as that in vogue in their churches. At the time of their expulsion in 1810 the business went into private hands. The peculiar scroll-like embellishments of the rococo period are absent. This work, therefore, belongs to the period immediately precedent, styled, as before mentioned, the "Zopfzeit" period.

Figure 42 (from "A Text-book of the Apothecaries Act," by Karl Hagen, 1778) represents the laboratory of the court-pharmacy at Koenigsberg. The fire-place and distilling apparatus are particularly conspicuous, and in their construction approach modern appliances. Karl Hagen, who lived in the latter half of the eighteenth century, superintended this laboratory, and was professor of physics and chemistry at the university. Beside the "Text-book of the Apothecaries Art," of which eight editions were published, he wrote "The Elements of Experimental

Chemistry," and "The Fundamental Principles of Chemistry."
Hagen, therefore, exerted a great influence in the education of
the pharmacists of his time. The wide experience evident in
these works was no doubt gathered by him in the laboratory
here pictured.

The practice of pharmacy in the eighteenth century was by
no means as remunerative as has been asserted. Its field was as
much invaded by grocers, spice dealers, distillers, etc., as it

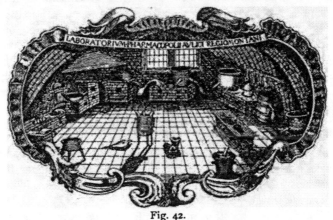

Fig. 42.

LABORATORY OF COURT PHARMACY AT KOENIGSBERG, A. D. 1778.

now is by notion dealers, etc. The archives of the Nuremburg
Collegii Pharmaceutici are encumbered with memorials respect-
ing the grievances of the apothecaries and the replies of the
accused thereto. These memorials are, as a rule, only a reca-
pitulation of similar complaints cited in preceding centuries.
In some instances the druggists suffered pecuniary losses from
causes entirely of their own creation. One was the habit of
sending New Year's presents to physicians and to customers,
which had grown to such proportions that the government interfered. The Anspach Gazette, November 23, 1796, contains this
announcement :

Since the practice among apothecaries of giving New Year's gifts to physicians and patients has been extensively abused, it should forthwith be discontinued. Apothecaries are therefore forbidden under severe penalty to continue
this destructive and demoralizing practice. This order is herewith made known
to the general public.   THE SECRETARY OF STATE AND WAR.

Nov. 16, 1796.

Although the eighteenth century pharmacists, more than ever before, were intent upon surrounding themselves with a scientific halo, and dubbed their apprentices "Discipuli," and the journeyman clerks "Subjecti," their education was still rudimentary, and but few possessed scientific attainments. A thorough knowledge of the natural sciences was not demanded, and what they knew was limited to what could be acquired in every-day experiences. The renowned Fr. Hoffman, who was professor at Halle from 1694 to 1743, in defining what knowledge the apothecary should possess, says : "The apothecary should know that an acid and an alkali, when brought in contact, will effervesce. It will suffice if he but know the effect, although he may be ignorant of the cause." Unflattering as Hoffman's assertion may seem, he was in the main correct in his premises. The learned apothecary, Trommsdorf, of Erfurt, takes a similar view of the state of pharmacy in the eighteenth century. Speaking of his apprenticeship, he says : " Rarely did I find men that approached my ideal. More frequently, on the other hand, I met with incompetency and slovenliness. Seldom, even, did I find a proper appreciation of the pharmacist's important calling by the general public. Pharmacy was almost universally looked upon as a trade, and the pharmacist as a mere tradesman. This fact pained me the more, the firmer I became convinced that pharmacy is a worthy branch of the natural sciences, and its devotees deserve the honors so freely bestowed on workers in other departments of the sciences. But how few of the druggists themselves were permeated by the importance of their calling !"

The recognition of this deplorable state of affairs induced Trommsdorf to employ all his powers in the furtherance of the art of pharmacy. In 1794 he published a pharmacal journal, and in 1795 founded a chemico-pharmacal institute, which met "a long felt want," since the universities were not yet supplied with laboratories adapted to the requirements of pharmacists. The studies in this institute embraced logic, mathematics, physics, botany, zoology, mineralogy, chemistry and pharmacy. Thus an opportunity was offered for the study of the branches of pharmacy which are at the present day a part of the universities. The result of this innovation was to lift pharmacy from its humble sphere and elevate it to the dignity of a scientific profession. Many apothecaries of the eighteenth century gained renown in the field of the sciences, in evidence of which the names of Ehrhart, Funk, Hudson, Geoffroy, Marggraf, Scheele, Weigleb, etc., etc., may be cited. They belonged to the apothecary's class, and will always be remembered in connection with chemistry and botany. The question, at times propounded, whether these men acquired their prominence because of their having been pharmacists, or in spite of or independent of this fact, can hardly be answered in a manner which will redound to the credit of pharmacy.

Dr. Dover, the inventor of Dover's powder, had been educated as an apothecary, and was a great friend and pupil of Sydenham. He began practice in Bristol, England, but despite his drug-store adjunct to practice, did not make a great financial success. Some merchants fitted out privateers, which were very successful in taking Spanish ships. He sailed with them as physician, and on February 2, 1708, visited Juan Fernandez, where he found and brought away Alexander Selkirk, the original of "Robinson Crusoe." In 1711 he began practice in London, and apothecaries and patients consulted him at the Jerusalem Coffee House. The originator of Fowler's solution, Thomas Fowler, of Stratford, was born in 1736. He also had been educated as an apothecary. Dr. Steer, the introducer of opodeldoc, a native of England, was a prominent apothecary of the eighteenth century.

In Ireland, during this period, the metrology was exceedingly confused ; troy weight and avoirdupois were both used by apothecaries, and many complaints resulted.

The social status of the pharmacist in some of the American provinces during the early part of the eighteenth century is shown by the enumeration of Jas. Tagree among the prominent citizens of New York City, in 1703, as an apothecary. The only other legally recognized apothecary in the province of New York, for a number of years, was Governor Hunter, who presided over the destinies of the colony for the decade, ending 1719. The Van Burens soon after began the practice of pharmacy in New York. They had, as early as 1706, practised pharmacy in New Brunswick, N. J., and Philadelphia. Their preparation, "The Red Drop," retained its reputation late into the nineteenth century.

John Johnstone practiced pharmacy at Perth Amboy early in the eighteenth century. He was very active in public service, and occupied several important positions. Some of his descendants still continue to practice pharmacy.

The first patent medicine was called "Tuscarora Rice," sold as a "consumption cure," by a Mrs. Masters, in 1711, and had a wide-spread reputation. She erected a large manufactory, and probably inaugurated the patent medicine trade in the United States. Indian medicine men of the "Sagwa" variety, and other traveling quacks, perambulated the country, selling worthless decoctions. These were stopped in New Jersey, in 1772, by a law passed at the instance of the State Medical Society which had been established in 1766. This law prohibited practice by mountebank doctors, or the sale of drugs or medicines by them. Under this act most of the drug-stores were run by licensees. The general merchants sold the crude drugs, and not infrequently came into conflict with the law.

Among the prominent practitioners of pharmacy in this century was the Rev. Jonathan Dickinson, of Elizabethtown, N. J., who wrote on the preparation of the ordinary vegetable drugs of America for medicinal use. Dr. Lawrence Vanderveer, of Millstone, N. J., was another pharmacist who gained celebrity by his introduction of scutellaria into medicine. Mr. Robert Eastburn, of New Brunswick, published a pharmacal work entitled a "Collection of Receipts," in 1755.

Later in the century, the mental activity consequent on the American Revolution resulted in the publication of the works of Schoepf and Barton on Materia Medica, and the publication, in 1778, of an army pharmacopœia under the auspices of Dr. Tilton, of Delaware. Salmon's "Herbal," the Dispensatory of Duncan, the Materia Medica of Lewis, long continued to be the chief text books. The influence of Salmon's "Herbal" was undoubtedly stimulating to the study of botany. From it Dr. Cadwallader Colden, the pharmacist-physician governor of New York, received the stimulus which led to his botanical studies, afterward so commended by Linnæus.

That there was great enthusiasm manifested in the study of the indigenous vegetable materia medica is obvious from the writings of Dr. Benjamin Rush, who anticipates that therefrom will result cures of many diseases. These botanical studies, in no small degree, brought about the disuse of the lancet.

The merchants who sold crude drugs were much addicted to adulteration, and one of them, Carnes of New York, is stated by Dr. Francis to have sold colored sawdust for rhubarb.

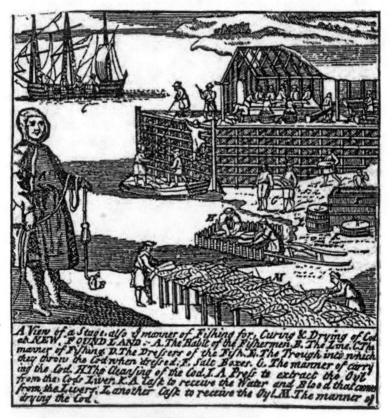

(From Keith's " Virginia," 1738).

Cod-liver oil began to assume a very prominent part in the armamentarium of American pharmacy in this century.

Ancient Distilling Apparatus.

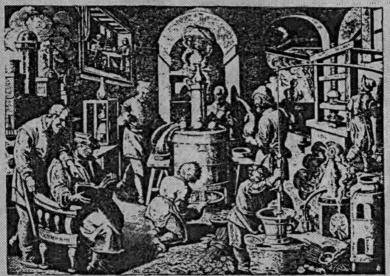

DISTILLATIO.
In igne situs omnium, arte, corporum   Vigens sit vndis, limpida et potissima.

Fig. 43.
(From a Copper-Print, 16th Century).

"Now 'tis evaporated and invisible,
  And upward flies, whence its airy source,
  Then to the earth returns again,
  That first unto it gave birth.
  Even so we live and die,
  Now bound, and now as vapor fly."
                                        —GOETHE.

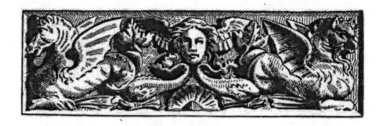

Chapter Six.

Ancient Distilling Apparatus.

ISTILLATION—the process by which volatile substances are separated from those of a more fixed
character—does not appear to have been much
practiced by the early Greeks and Romans. The
earliest reference made to it we trace to Synesius,
who, about 410 B. C., was Bishop of Ptolemais.* The Arabian
Galen, "Rhazes of Bagdad," likens the process of distillation to
the condition in nasal catarrh. "The stomach," he says,"is the
kettle, the head is the cap, and the nose is the conducting and
cooling tube, from which the product of distillation drips."
From this we learn that the public must have been quite familiar
with the process, and, in fact, we find it frequently referred to in
Arabian medical works.

In the thirteenth century, Furno of Basel, Thaddaus of Florence, and Arnoldus of Villanova, were largely instrumental in
introducing the products of distillation into the occidental materia medica, which effort was particularly successful in the case
of brandy and alcohol. These were very soon extensively used
as a beverage, so that about the year A. D. 1500, laws were deemed
necessary in several European states to counteract by legal restrictions the growing tendency to over-indulgence. The law of
Nuremburg decreed that brandy should neither be sold in shops
nor in the open market-place on Sundays or other holidays.

The increasing consumption of spirits, and the consequent
multiplication of distilled medicinal waters, are abundant proof
that the art of distilling had made considerable progress in the

* Kopp, History of Chemistry. (79)

fifteenth century.   Hieronymus Brunschwyck gives us a very lucid
description of the apparatus in use in his day, in "The New
Book on the Art of Distilling," and "The Art of Distilling Composite Things," both richly illustrated with wood-cuts.   We have
drawn largely on these books for our information.

The first book was published on the 8th of May, 1500, and
the other a few years later.   At that time the word "distil," "to
drip," had a wider application than at the present day.

What in modern times is known as maceration, digestion,
filtration, percolation and extraction, were all embraced under
the head of distillation.   Before the distillation proper of any
substance was attempted, it was first subjected to a process of
digestion in a glass retort for purposes of solution and softening.
A great variety of methods were employed to obtain the requi-
site degree of warmth.   One primitive method is thus described :
"In a convenient locality, preferably in a cellar, a pit five feet
deep was excavated.   This was partially filled with a layer of
unslaked lime ; upon this followed a layer of horse manure,
whereupon the vessel with the material was brought into place,
and the whole covered up with another liberal supply of horse
dung.   The lime was then slaked by the pouring on of lukewarm
water, thereby establishing a sort of fermentation, and an elevated
temperature, which was maintained for several days, whereupon
the substances in the pit were renewed, and the process repeated
as often as found expedient."   The simpler method of digesting
matter by the aid of the sun or heat from a stove was also resorted
to.   To augment the sun's heat concave mirrors were employed.
The digesting retort was placed between one of these and the
sun, so as to receive the direct rays, and also the reflected heat
from the mirror.

Other peculiar methods, resorted to in the Middle Ages for
securing an elevated temperature in the process of digestion, consisted in placing the vessels in ant-hills, in bread, ashes, in a
water-bath, etc.   For digesting in bread, the vessel was packed
in dough, placed in an oven and baked like ordinary bread.
The forms of the vessels employed were as varied as the methods
for securing the required elevation of temperature.   Particular
stress was laid upon the importance of choosing such vessels as
favored the return of the condensed vapors to the bottom of the

vessel, so that the fluids could again penetrate the macerating substance, and thus repeatedly make the circuit.

The following illustrations, taken from the works of Brunsch-wyck, show us a number of these vessels:

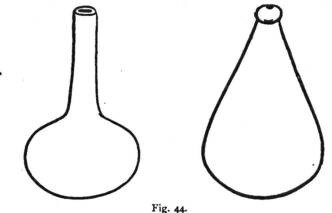

Fig. 44.

a, VIAL, SIXTEENTH CENTURY.   *b,* CUCURBITE.

Fig. 44 *a,* was known as a vial.   Fig. 44 *b,* was called a cucur-bite from its resemblance to the shape of a gourd.

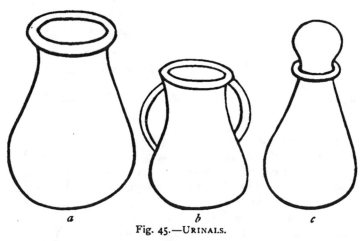

a   *b*   *c*

Fig. 45.—URINALS.

Figs. 45 *a, b* and *c,* represent a variety of urinals.   Fig. 46 *a* and *b,* are simple circulatories; *c,* a circulatory with lateral

beak ; *d*, a double circulatory, and *e*, a pelican circulatory, with
two conducting tubes for the returning fluid.

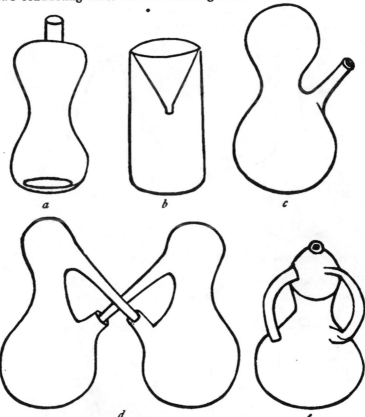

Fig. 46 *a*, *b*, *c*, *d* and *e*.—Circulatories.

The funnels of the Middle Ages were, likewise,
somewhat differently shaped than at present, as
shown in the figure. Brunschwyck says they were
used to separate oil and water and for conveying acids
from one vessel into another. They were probably
not used in the clarifying of liquids, since the process
of filtering through paper had not been introduced. In
his time liquids were clarified by running them through
a linen or woolen bag, or they were "distilled per

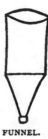

Funnel.

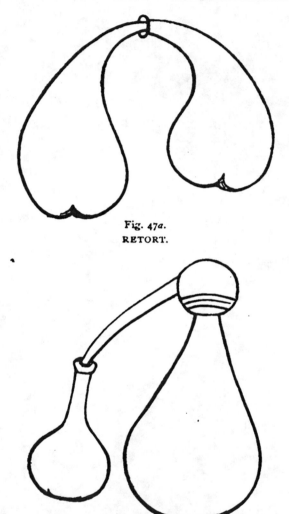

Fig. 47*a*.
RETORT.

Fig. 47*b*.
THE ALEMBIC.

filtram." This process consisted in placing the liquid to be clarified in a bowl or pan, and connecting it with a vessel on a lower plane by means of a strip of felt or woolen cloth. By virtue of the capillary action of these bodies, the fluid was

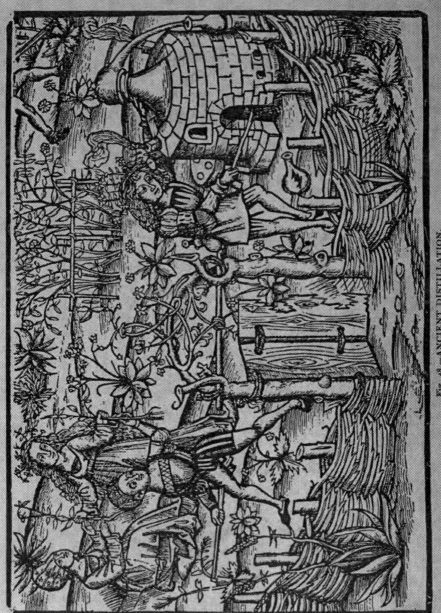

Fig. 48.—ANCIENT DISTILLATION.

carried over and dripped into the lower vessel. In the case of very volatile substances two retorts were used, the beak of the lower one being cemented into that of the higher one, see Fig. 47*a*. The liquid was then carried over by the strip of felt which had previously been properly adjusted on the inside of the retorts.

The most ancient form of distilling apparatus was probably the alembic, from the Greek, meaning "a cover;" and the Arabian article "al," originally applied to the head of a still only. The alembic was placed on an earthen vessel or glass cucurbite, and cemented to the latter, and after a receiver had been adjusted to the beak of the alembic, this primitive distilling apparatus was complete in all its details. Fig. 47*b*.

In Fig. 48 we see one of these apparatus in use, placed on an ordinary distilling stove. Although the distillation is pictured as taking place in a garden, it is not probable that it was practiced in the open air, exposed to wind and weather. It is well known that the artists of the Middle Ages not only sought to emphasize the minutest details of the objects pictured, but they also attempted to demonstrate their association with the objects in nature, by placing these in juxtaposition, no matter how much out of place the one or the other might be, and without apparently ever being aware of the impropriety of such an arrangement. The plant world was, as we have seen, the main source of medicinal waters, and in the distillation of the latter women frequently took part. Hence the artist places the apparatus in a garden in which, beside the two apothecaries, are two women engaged in gathering plants; all these details serving to indicate that the object of the distillation was the gaining of medicinal waters. The glass still-heads known as alembics were made in a variety of styles.

The early alembic had the great fault that it allowed the vapors that condensed on its surface to flow back into the vessel too readily, thus greatly retarding the process, Fig. 49*a*. This defect was remedied by making a groove on the inside wall, and near the neck of the alembic, Fig. 49*b*, with which the opening into the beak was continuous. Thus the condensed liquid collected in this groove and was conducted to the beak, toward which the groove was slightly inclined.

The lack of a cooling apparatus was a very serious obstacle

to a successful and profitable distillation, on account of the escape of large quantities of uncondensed vapors. To obviate this in a measure, and to gain a larger cooling surface, the alembics were constructed in the shape of tall cones (see Fig. 49*c*), and were made of glazed earthenware, copper, zinc or lead, and

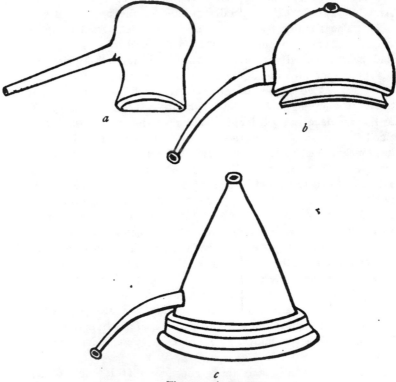

Fig. 49.—ALEMBICS.

placed over shallow vessels of like material. This style was mostly used for the distilling of water.

The Middle Age retorts were, on account of their impracticable shape, adapted only to such liquids that during ebullition did not escape through the beak. Their use for distilling purposes was therefore limited, and found application mostly for the "distillation per filtram," before described, and for purposes of digestion. To render the distilling vessels, which were in greater part made of glass, more resisting to the heat of an open fire, they were encased in a mass composed of clay, hemp-hatchel, horse-dung and wine. This mass was applied to the depth of one-half inch and allowed to dry. If, in spite of this precaution,

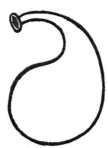

the vessel should crack, a cloth, spread with a putty of red-lead, lime, flour and the white of egg, was placed over the fissure. The cloth used for this purpose was previously saturated with salt water and white of egg to render it fire-proof. For cementing the still-heads to the container and the receiving vessel to the former, a variety of pastes were in use. When a high degree of temperature was required, the so-called Lutum sapientiæ was used. This cement was composed of

Middle Age Retort.

clay, horse-dung, ground brick, ground iron, salt water and white of egg. When a lesser temperature sufficed, a paste composed of starch and soaked paper was applied.

Common retorts served as receivers, but in case of very volatile substances, vessels with a lateral beak were substituted (see Fig. 50). In consequence of the constantly increasing consumption of spirits, the small glass apparatus could no longer supply the demand, and gradually the copper kettles, not very unlike our modern apparatus (Fig.

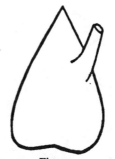

Fig. 50.

51), came into use. To condense the vapors, the still-head was made in the shape of a so-called "Moor's head," being surmounted by a copper mantel which was filled with cold water.

For the purpose of rectification, the spirit was repeatedly and slowly distilled through a head without the customary furrow, the lower orifice of the head having been plugged with a sponge saturated in oil. The water, which was vaporized simultaneously with the alcohol, was condensed on the sponge, whilst the alcohol vapors passed through the pores of the sponge, and after being condensed in the cooling apparatus, escaped into the receiver. To obtain an alcohol of a still higher percentage, an apparatus

is described in Figure 52, which may be considered as a fore-
runner of those in use at the present day.   Here we see the retort
connected with a worm-like tube that repeatedly passes through
a larger upright tube filled with cold water.   The vapor, as it

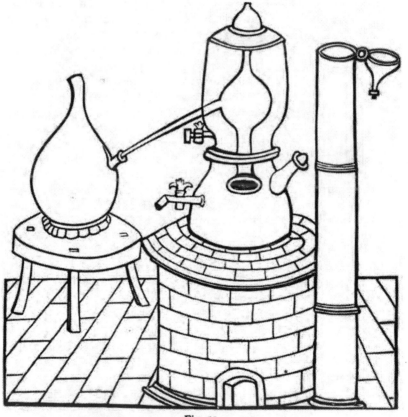

Fig. 51.
DISTILLING APPARATUS.

rises in this tube, experiences an insufficient refrigeration, and
the more volatile alcohol, finding its way to the remotest coil,
finally condenses and reaches the receptacle ; whereas the water,
which condenses earlier, finds its way back to the kettle or retort.
That Basilius Valentinus had, in the fifteenth century, advised
the use of tartrate of potassa for the dehydration of alcohol, is

no doubt known to the reader, and needs but incidentally to be
recalled here. An exact determination of its strength was impossible before the discovery of the alcoholometer at the close

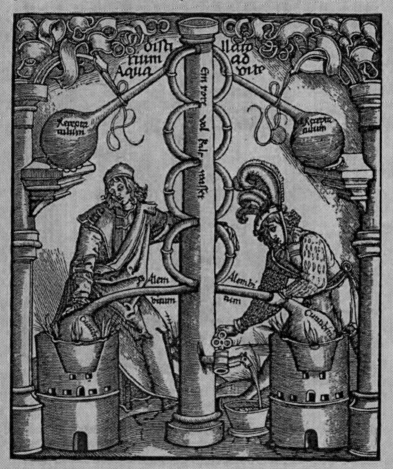

Fig. 52.
IMPROVED DISTILLING APPARATUS.

of the eighteenth century. Brunschwyck thought he had
obtained spirits of the highest possible percentage, when a linen
cloth saturated with it would also be destroyed after the alcohol
had been ignited and entirely consumed. In case of very

hydrous alcohol the remaining water, of course, protected the linen from the flame. Another test consisted in dropping olive oil into the spirits; if the oil sank to the bottom, the alcohol was proof. Since the specific gravity of olive oil is 0.915 an alcohol of sixty per cent. met this requirement. In place of the linen test, we later find mention of the powder test. Powder saturated with alcohol of proper strength should burn with a puff after the

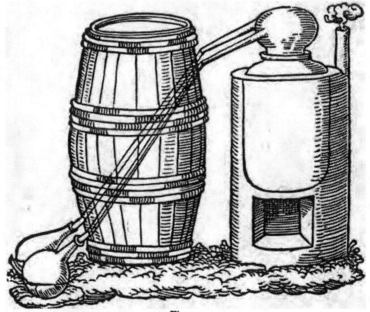

Fig. 53.
DISTILLING APPARATUS, 1560.

alcohol had been consumed. Albertus Magnus has called attention to the fact that distillates from metal apparatus frequently carry with them metallic impurities, and, based on this authority, Brunschwyck also warns against the indiscriminate use of such apparatus. The Nuremburg apothecary ordinance of June 7, 1555, entirely forbids their employment in drug-stores. This order was, however, soon found to overreach itself as applied to pharmacy, and in the ordinances of 1592 we find no more mention of it. In the Middle Ages distilling by druggists had been

limited to medicinal waters, but when in the sixteenth century
they entered upon the distilling of more volatile subtances, they
felt the need of adopting the cooling apparatus already in use in
distilleries. The books of the latter half of the sixteenth century
that treat on this subject, show that just about this time the greatest improvements were being made in the line of cooling appliances.

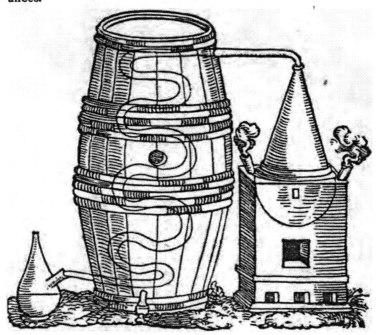

Fig. 54.

"The Distiller's Book," by G. Ryff, 1567, furnishes a number
of illustrations bearing on this subject. In Fig. 53, the cap has
two conducting pipes that pass obliquely through a barrel filled
with water. Ryff acknowledges that for distilling larger quantities
this apparatus is entirely unsatisfactory, and in its place recommends the apparatus shown in Fig. 54. Fig. 55 represents an
apparatus used in France at this time. In connection with the
renewal of the water in the cooling apparatus, the fact that the
warmer water rises to the surface and the cooler water collects

in the lower part of the vessel, appears to have been entirely over-looked or was not understood.   In comparing the apparatus here

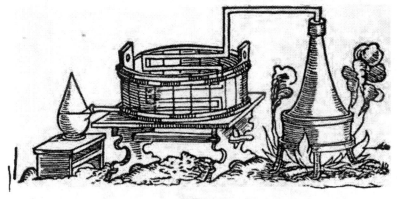

Fig. 55.
APPARATUS IN USE IN FRANCE IN 1560.

pictured with those of modern construction, we therefore miss in the former the afferent tube for conveying the cold water to the base of the tub, and the effer-ent tube for conveying away the heated surface-water.   To secure, by one and the same operation, both the pure or more volatile and the more sluggish product, an apparatus like the one shown in Fig. 56 was used.   The helm was sup-plied with two conducting tubes, each of which was continuous with a groove around the inner wall of the helm, on the plane of their division.

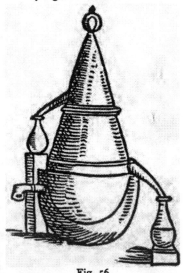

Fig. 56.

Fig. 57 shows a section of a stove and apparatus used in process for dry distillation, per descensum.   The stove was divided into two compartments by a diaphragmatic contrivance, into a central opening of which an earthen vessel was cemented from below. The mouth of this vessel, which opened into the upper half of the stove, was covered over by a piece of perforated tin. Over this a similar vessel, previously filled with the substance to be distilled, was inverted, and the mouths of the two pots carefully adjusted. A fire was then started around the upper pot, causing the products of distillation, the heavy tar oils, to drip through the holes in the tin into the lower vessel, where they could be secured by means of a conducting tube at the bottom of the pot. For want of a stove the

Fig. 57.

lower pot was frequently sunk into the ground and a fire started around the upper one, when the same object was attained. The oleum juniperi empyreumaticum was prepared in this manner.

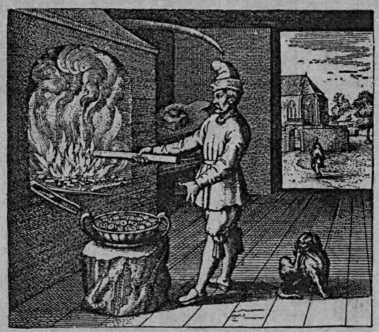

Fig. 58.
ALCHEMIST'S FIRE-PLACE, 1618.

"What friend is like the might of fire,
    When men can watch and wield the ire?
    Whate'er we shape or work, we owe
    Still to that heaven-descended glow."

—SCHILLER (The Lay of the Bell).

Chapter Seven.

Early Chemico-Pharmacal Fire-Places and Stoves.

THE important office assigned to fire in the labors of alchemists — the precursors of the modern chemists—early led to the construction of special hearths and stoves, by which the heat required in the practice of the hermetic art could be conveniently supplied and regulated. As early as the ninth century the Arabian "Geber," who lived in Seville, wrote a work which has come down to us in the Latin version, as "De Fornacibus Construendis," in which he describes stoves for calcinating, melting and distilling.

As a result of the advancement of pharmacy in the occidental countries after the twelfth century, the principles underwent vast changes and improvements. The principal stoves in use in the Middle Ages for the preparation of medicines, and in particular those used in the process of distilling, are minutely described in the two books by Hieronymus Brunschwyck, referred to in the preceding chapter. In Figure 48, Chapter Six, a stove of the most simple construction is shown. This class of stoves was built of brick or glazed tile, that could be readily taken apart and readjusted. On one side, at the base, was an aperture for the introduction of fuel and the removal of ashes, and on either side were lesser openings for draught purposes. On the other side of the stove, opposite the main aperture, were two openings for the escape of the smoke. When distilling from a fire-proof kettle, this was placed directly over the open fire in an opening left in the top of the stove. But in case glass, earthen or lead vessels were employed, the distillation

(97)

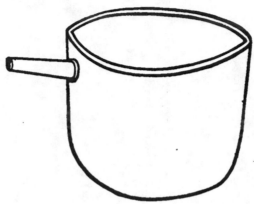

Fig. 59.
FIRE KETTLE.

was proceeded with either "per cinerem" or "per arenam."
To this end ashes or sand were spread two or three inches deep
on an iron or stone plate, with which the opening in the top of

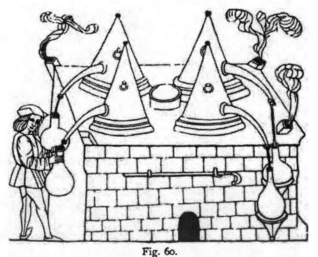

Fig. 60.
DISTILLERY HEARTH.

the stove had been closed, and upon this the distilling vessel
was placed.   To distil with the aid of a water bath, "per balneum
mariæ," this simple stove was turned into a so-called coppel

stove, by cementing a copper kettle into the opening in place of the plate which had before served as a cover. This was called a "coppel," and was filled with water, into which the distilling vessel was placed. To keep the latter in position it was weighted above and below with leaden rings. To protect the hot stones from injury by water, which might escape during ebullition, the copper kettle was ordinarily supplied with a lateral pipe to conduct the overflow to a safe distance. Fig. 59.

For the purpose of carrying on several distillations on the same fire, the so-called distilling hearths (Fig. 60) were devised, constructed of baked or sundried brick. These hearths were divided into an upper and a lower compartment by means of a grate. In the

Fig. 61.
COPPEL HEARTH.

lower part was an opening for the removal of the ashes, and for allowing air to reach the fuel above the grate. The fuel was introduced through an opening in the centre of the iron plate covering the stove. The smoke escaped through holes left at the corners. To regulate the fire, some of these holes were closed by means of earthen plugs. The iron plate was partially covered by tiles, leaving open spaces at intervals that were filled up with sand, upon which the distilling vessels were placed.

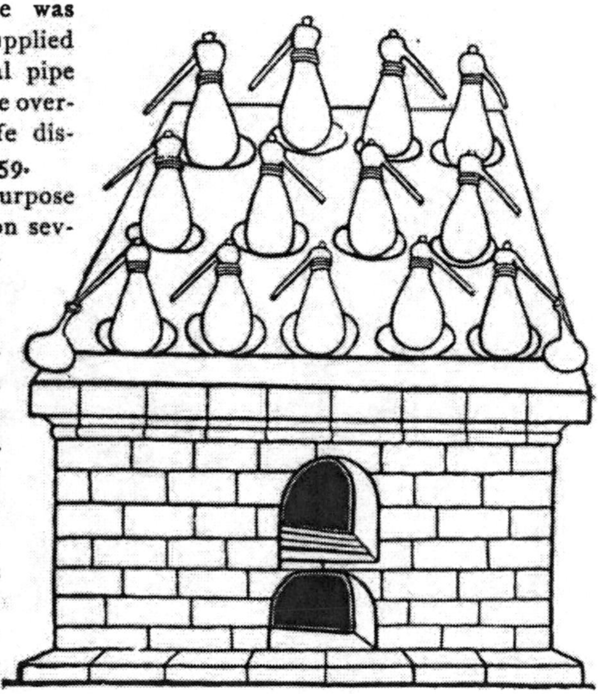

In Fig. 60 we see four distilling pans placed in these sand-baths, and surmounted by the tall condensing caps spoken of in a former chapter. To utilize one fire to the utmost, these hearths were made of large dimensions, frequently with ten to thirty coppels. These coppels were not made of copper, as in the case of the water-bath described above, but of clay, on account of its greater cheapness and resistance to fire. Fig. 61 shows us one of these coppel hearths with thirteen stills covered by alembics. When the process of distillation was begun a receiver was, of course, attached to the beak of each alembic, as shown in con-

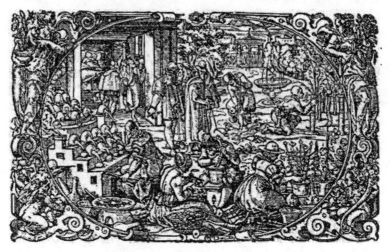

Fig. 62.
DISTILLING SCENE, A. D. 1592.

nection with two of them in the illustration.   These coppel hearths somewhat resemble the galley stoves of our chemical factories ; the latter being so named from the fact, that when fully equipped with retorts, their appearance calls to mind the row of oars protruding from a galley.   In Fig. 62, which is taken from "The New Medicine Book," by Jacob Theodor Tabernæ-montanus, published at Neustadt in 1592, is seen a distilling apparatus, set up in a garden.   In this case the hearth is arranged terrace-like.   From a description of the process we learn, that "Numerous copper or earthen vessels are placed upon the hearth ; they are then filled with the fresh comminuted herbs, which have been saturated with water or wine. Over each vessel is turned a beaked cap, and the small vessels receive the water as it drops from the beaks."

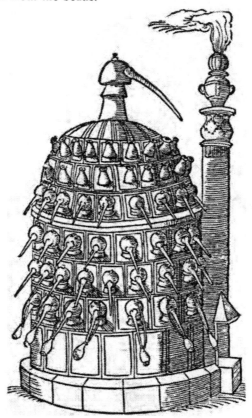

Fig. 63.
DISTILLING STOVE, A. D. 1586.

In the "Herb-Book" of Matthiolus, published in 1586, a somewhat similar stove is pictured and described, Fig. 63, in which the vessels placed on the stove, as in the preceding picture, are superseded by the tiles themselves, made in imitation of jars, as is plainly seen in the two upper rows depicted in Fig. 63. Matthiolus, in describing this stove, says it "is

extensively used at Venice. The distillation proceeds quickly
and satisfactorily, for in twenty-four hours it will distil over 100
pounds of water. The stove is built round, and is made by a
potter, just as he would any other tile stove or hearth that we

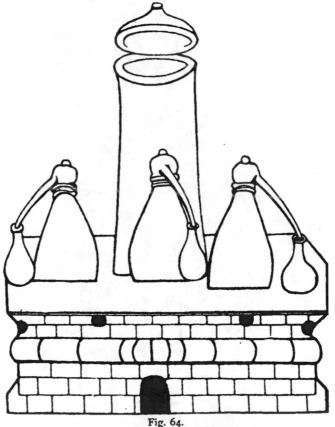

Fig. 64.

ALTHANOR DISTILLING STOVE.

use in our homes. The hollow tiles encircle the stove in a number of layers, and are glazed and shaped almost like urinal
glasses. These tiles are capped by glass distilling helms, which
are simply turned over them. The receivers are attached to the
beaks, and held in place by strings that are tied to the knob on
the helm. Now, when one wishes to distil, a fire is started in the

stove, but the plants or flowers are not yet put into the tile vessels, for the excessive heat would destroy their properties. It is, therefore, better to wait until the maximum heat has subsided. Then, when the stove is reasonably hot, it is closed tightly, so that it may retain an equable temperature as long as possible. Now you may introduce the plants and flowers into the cavities, turn the glass helms over them, and allow the distillation to proceed. The resulting distillate will be much finer than that obtained by means of zinc vessels."

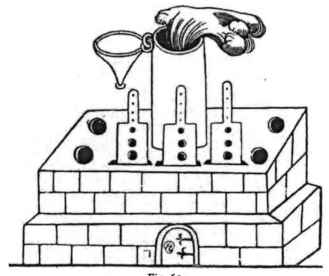

Fig. 65.
"WIND" DISTILLING STOVE.

For tedious and protracted fire operations the so-called lazy "Heintz"* or "Althanor" (from αϑανατος, everlasting, immortal) was the most desirable and serviceable heating apparatus. The distinguishing feature of this stove was a tall pipe, Fig. 64, closed at the top by a cover, containing the fuel, which, as in the modern American stoves, gradually found its way down to the grate to take the place of the fuel consumed. These hearths were usually supplied with three or four coppels, and each of these with its own fire-place, which was connected with the pipe

*A corruption of the word "Heinrich."

furnishing the fuel. Each fire-place had an opening, controlled
by a register, for the escape of the smoke. By the manipulation
of these registers and the closing of the ash-ports the fire was
regulated. For the distillation of many pharmaceutical preparations the highest degree of temperature, consistent with complete
control over the operation, was required. To effect this it was
found necessary to be able to regulate the supply of air. These
features were embodied in greatest perfection in the "Wind-
stove," Fig. 65. A powerful draught was established by means

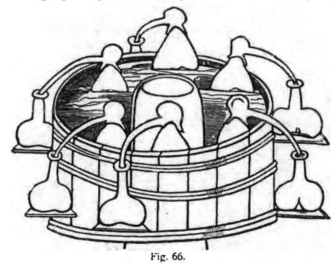

Fig. 66.
DISTILLING APPARATUS.

of a stove-pipe, as at the present day. The pipe served for the
introduction of fuel and for the escape of the smoke. The fire-
place could be shut off from the flue by these registers, and in
addition the draft could be entirely suppressed by means of a
cover on the pipe, so that the fire was at all time under absolute
control. To utilize the great amount of heat constantly going
to waste, Brunschwyck describes a device, Fig. 66, which, on
account of its complicated nature, was probably not often
resorted to, and should rather be classed with the other numerous technical playthings of the Middle Ages. It consisted in
extending the stove-pipe to an upper floor in the house, and
then guiding it through a wooden tub filled with water. The

pipe imparted enough heat to the water to make this available for digestion and the distillation of very volatile substances. For creating an intense heat to melt metals, without resorting to a blast, Brunschwyck describes a stove constructed on the same plan as the modern wind-stove. But while the modern wind-stove usually consists of a sheet-iron mantel, lined with fire-proof cement, the Middle Age stove, as seen in Fig. 67, is con-

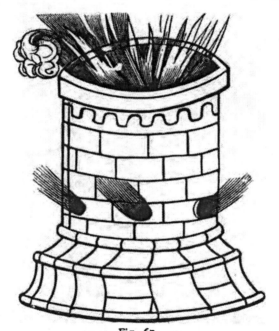

Fig. 67.
MIDDLE AGE STOVE.

structed of wedge-shaped tiles, like those now frequently used in the construction of wells and chimneys. As in the modern stove, the interior was divided by a grate, underneath which, in the walls of the stove, numerous air holes were left. The fuel consisted of wood or charcoal, and the metal to be melted was packed into a crucible and placed in the fire.

Since in many instances the proximity of the fire proved to be a disturbing element in the calcinating and melting processes, a stove was desired in which the substance could be subjected to a high degree of heat without bringing it in contact with the flame. One of these stoves, known as 'a "reverberatory" furnace, is shown in Figure 68.   At the junction of the lower with the middle third is a grate for the support of the fire.   The substance to be operated upon were placed in a separate chamber, against which the flames were directed, and upon which, by a special flue arrangement, they were deflected or reverberated on passing from the fire-chamber to the chimney.   Brunschwyck recom-

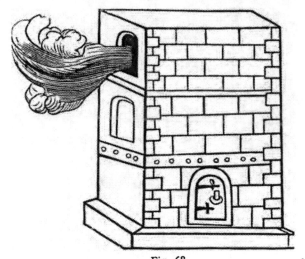

Fig. 68.
REVERBERATORY FURNACE.

mends this stove for making gold powder, which, according to his method, was effected by melting together gold and mercury, triturating the amalgam and then driving out the mercury by heating the compound in the reverberatory furnace. These stoves naturally found more application in metallurgical processes than in pharmacal manipulations.

Besides enumerating tan-bark, wood and charcoal, Ryff, in 1567, also mentions mineral coal for fuel, which he declares to be of inestimable value to alchemists. He draws a comparison between the living heat produced by these substances, and the artificial heat by which the activity of nature is imitated, which latter in the interior of the earth heats the waters that rise to the surface, and furnish us with the wonderful natural springs for the cure of disease. "To imitate this heat," he says, "take one part of fresh, hot unslaked lime, one-half part sulphur, one-quarter part saltpetre and one-eighth part nice clean alum. Powder each ingredient separately and promptly mix them. Put them into a brass globe, which is then closed, so as to insure the contents against the action of air and water. It is then placed in a tub of water. The steam from the warm lime will attach itself to the inner wall of the globe, and will be resolved into drops by the action of the cold water on the outside of the globe, which drops, in their turn, will be attracted by the alum. This moisture, with the inherent moisture of the alum, will cause the latter to melt, whereupon the lime will become very hot and burn. To maintain its ardor the saltpetre has been added to furnish it with air, and the sulphur to supply it with nourishment, without which two conditions no fire can be maintained. If you prepare this self-heating globe with scrupulous care, you may derive great benefit from it, for if you make it large enough you can heat a large tub of water with it, and thus secure a kind of natural heating bath, similar to the hot springs."

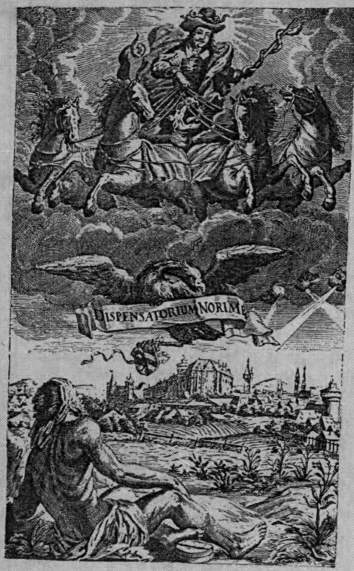

Fig. 69.
(From Title-page of Pharmacopœia of 1666).
(109)

" O, mickle is the powerful grace that lies,
    In herbs, plants, stones, and their true qualities!
    For nought so vile that on the earth doth live,
    But to the earth some special good doth give."

—ROMEO AND JULIET

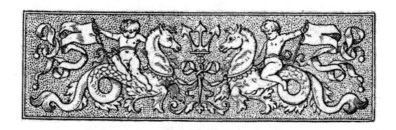

Chapter Eight.

Ancient Pharmacopœias.

ONSIDERING that the cuneiform inscriptions contain formularies corresponding, in some respects, to the modern idea of a Pharmacopœia, the earliest collection of formulas, showing evidence of supervision over drugs, was the "Prayogamrita" of Vardy-achin-tamani, a Sanscrit work. The "Compositiones Medica" of Scribonius Longus, written 42 A. D., is evidence of a Roman attempt to fix some standard.

About 900 A. D. appeared the "Ibdal," an Arabian book of formulas, which gave directions as to the preparation of drugs. Under the influence of this Arabic training, the school founded at Salerno in the seventh century, with an academy founded at Naples in the eleventh century, long maintained an enviable reputation. Through the influence of these schools, drug-stores, called "Stationares," were established throughout Italy. In the first medical ordinance for Naples and Sicily, under Frederic II, the apothecaries were directed to be governed by the "Antidotarium" of Nicolaus, the superintendent of the medical school at Salerno. This Dispensatory contains about one hundred and fifty galenical preparations, alphabetically arranged, and gives a description of their medicinal properties, with directions for administration. This work, with the medical works of Avicenna, Serapion, Scribonius and others, formed a nucleus for more elaborate productions in the interest of the Apothecaries Guild.

A "formulary" of the eleventh century, now in the archives of Piedmont, is devoted, first, to receipts for making good ink and illuminative parchment. The vegetable remedies enumerated include aloes, camphor, cassia, lettuce, opium, rue, linseed, mustard, etc.   The formulary is largely based on the work of Lucius Apuleius Platonicus on the virtue of herbs.

The Antidotarium of Myrepsius was the authority in the thirteenth century.   The "Antidotarium Magnum seu Dispensatorium ad Aromatorios," extensively used in Italy, was published at Florence in 1498.   These Italian works were long recognized as the chief authorities elsewhere.   The study of the science in Italy gave an impetus to science all over Europe.

The sixteenth century was marked by the appearance of a number of pharmacopœias in the modern sense of the term. The Latin countries first began to exhibit evidences of an independence of the Italian yoke, for in 1543, Lyons established and published the "Pharmacopœia Lugdensis."*   In southern Germany the sixteenth century was the golden era.   The arts and sciences were being cultivated by men like Dürer, Vischer and Krafft.   The reformatory spirit of the age was shown in the field of medicine, by the enactment of rational medical laws.   Apothecaries' ordinances, dating from the earliest days of the century, were supplemented by one enacted in 1529 by the Nuremburg Senate, which, among other things, fixed methods for the preparation of medicines.   One extract reads :

All the Laxativa, such as Electuaria and Pillulæ, must be prepared and dispensed by the druggists in accordance with the directions in the book known as the Luminare majus.   To avoid any error or oversight in the preparation of these Laxativa, and to insure even preparations by all druggists, these Laxativa have been carefully copied from the Luminare majus by the doctors of medicine. Each druggist will be furnished with a copy, by which he must be guided, to the exclusion of all other formulas.

The "Luminare majus" was a collection of formula from the later Greek, Roman and Arabian medical works.   Its author, the Alexandrian Joh. Jac. Manlius de Bosco, added a lengthy explanation to each formula, thus making it rather a text-book than a pharmacopœia.   Strictly speaking, only one of the works hitherto mentioned deserves the title of pharmacopœia, as they were more like the ancient Egyptian formularies deciphered by Ebers, and the Assyrian translated by Sayce.   All, however, are of value in tracing the evolution of the pharmacopœia.

* Rice, Reference Handbook of the Medical Sciences.

The first work corresponding to the modern idea of a pharmacopœia, which received legal sanction in Europe, was the result of the labors of Valerius Cordus. This "Pharmacorum Conficiendorum Ratio, Vulgo Vocant Dispensatorium," was published without a date by John Petreyers at Nuremburg. Its author was born February 18, 1515, at Simtshausen, in Hesse. His father, Enricius Cordus, was professor of medicine at Marburg. Valerius and his brother entered the University very early, and received its baccalaureate degree in 1531. Valerius went to Wittenburg where he became a teacher. In 1543 he proceeded to Italy to study, and died at Rome, December 25, 1544. There are many contradictory reports in historical literature concerning his Dispensatory. The preface to the first edition states that "Valerius Cordus, the son of Enrich Cordus, while on his journey to Italy to assuage his thirst for knowledge, stopped at Nuremburg and was well received by its circle of learned men." He associated particularly with the physicians who, upon learning that he had carefully compiled a work containing all old and new medical preparations, with many improvements of his own, and that this book had been introduced in manuscript form in a number of cities in Saxony, requested him to furnish a copy for the Nuremburg druggists. Valerius, doubting that they would adopt his formulas without legal sanction, turned over his manuscript to the Senate for examination and approval. The Senate accepted it with thanks, and appointed a committee of physicians to investigate the formulas, so that in case changes were found necessary they could be made with the approval of the author. This committee declared it to be the best and most complete work of the kind extant. The Senate ordered it printed, and directed all druggists to prepare their medicines according to the directions therein laid down. The author died in Italy before the book was printed. It was published after his death by the High Senate of Nuremburg as "a lasting memorial to the learned and brilliant youth, Valerius Cordus."

The Dispensatory, which appeared in September, 1546, seems to have created quite a sensation, for even outside of Nuremberg it passed through numerous editions and reprints. The following are known: One Parisian in 1548; three Lyonaise, 1552,

1559 and 1599; two Venetian, 1556 and 1563, and one Antwerpian, 1580. The book, like all scientific works of the period, was printed in Latin. The names of the compounds were derived, in part, from the ingredients, in part from their properties, or, finally, from the name of the author. According to the first-mentioned method of nomenclature, a plaster which contained the juice of fenugreek, linseed and marshmallow, was called Emplastrum diachylon, "plaster with juice." A plaster containing vinegar and saffron was called Emplastrum oxycroceum, "sour saffron plaster." In the course of time these plasters underwent changes and improvements, and the substance to which the remedy owed its name was frequently omitted. The modern Emplastr. diachylon contains no juices, and the Emplastr. oxycroceum of to-day does not contain vinegar, and but infrequently saffron.

The names of many preparations by this modification in their preparation became problems for the philologist. The etymological obscurity of opodeldoc, which has become proverbial, is an instance. Its origin may be easily traced to the old opodeldoc plaster of the last Nuremburg edition of the "Dispensatorii Valerii Cordi." This does not contain any ingredients found in modern opodeldoc, but its then chief component parts were Opoponax, Bedellium and Aristolochi root. The first sylable of the first word, Opo- ; the second syllable of the second word, -del-, and the last syllable of the third word, -loch, gives Opodelloch, as Paracelsus wrote it, which became Opodeltoch, and finally, Opodeldoc. Simples are mentioned by Cordus only when special manipulation is required to render them serviceable as remedies.

The most important part of his book is a collection of receipts by Greek, Roman and Arabian physicians, by Dioscorides, of Sicily; Galenus, of Pergamus ; Andromachus, the body physician of Nero ; Rhazes, of Bagdad, " the Arabian Galen ; Avicenna ("Scheich el Reis," or "prince of physicians)"; Mesuë, the younger, and Nicolaus Præpositus, of Salerno. The formulary contained chiefly substances derived from the vegetable and animal kingdoms. The compounds were of a class known as Galenical preparations from the noted Roman physician, Claudius Galenus, who placed great faith in complex compounds.

The heterogeneous character of the innumerable ingredients of many of those compounds impress the modern mind with the idea that human life must have been greatly endangered by such remedies. It is easy to believe that Shakespere, a master in combining poetical fancy with devotion to fact, must have been acquainted with Cordus' work, for many of the latter's compounds recall the witch's broth in " Macbeth " :

" Round about the cauldron go ;
In the poisoned entrails throw.
Toad, that under cold stone
Days and nights has thirty-one
Swelter'd venom, sleeping got,
Boil them first i' the charmed pot.
Fillet of a fenny snake,
In the cauldron boil and bake ;
Eye of newt and toe of frog,
Wool of bat and tongue of dog,
Adder's fork and blind worm's sting,
Lizard's leg, and howlet's wing,
For a charm of powerful trouble,
Like a hell-broth boil and bubble.
Scale of dragon, tooth of wolf,
Witches' mummy, maw and gulf
Of the ravin'd salt-sea shark,
Root of hemlock, digg'd i' the dark,
Liver of blaspheming Jew,
Gall of goat, and slips of yew
Sliver'd i' the moon's eclipse,
Nose of Turk and Tartar's lips,
Finger of birth-strangled babe
Ditch-delivered by a drab,
Make the gruel thick and slab :
Add thereto a tiger's chaudron,
For the ingredients of our cauldron."

The preparations in Cordus' Dispensatory are divided into Aromatics, Opiates, Confections, Conserves, Purges, Pills, Syrups, Electuaries, Plasters, Cerates, Troches, Salves and Oils. There are additional directions for some few simples. Antidotes and disinfectants, classed with the opiates, appear to have been the main remedies in the time of Cordus. The principal representatives of these were the two electuaries, " Theriac " and " Mithridat." Both were originally intended as antidotes, but at a later day fallen into repute as remedies for contagious diseases.

Mithridat was a compound originally invented by Mithridates Eupator, King of Pontus, who lived in constant fear of poison, and studied toxicology by testing poisons on criminals, and taking poisons and their antidotes himself every day in the year. His system became so accustomed to the poisons, that when, on the day of his defeat by Pompey, he attempted to poison himself to avoid capture, the poison failed, and he ordered one of his soldiers to kill him. Among the papers of the defeated king, Pompey found the receipt for this electuary, which had a great reputation. This receipt, and other medical manuscripts found with the body, were translated by Pompey's freedman, the grammarian, Lenæus, into Latin. Thus, as Pliny * says, " Pompey benefited society no less than the state by his victory."

Originally the receipt for Mithridat was not very complicated, but was improved upon by Damocrates, the body physician of Nero. This improved formula, containing fifty-five ingredients, is introduced by Cordus in his Dispensatory. Andromachus, another body physician of Nero, still further improved upon the formula and increased its ingredients.

One of his principal additions was the flesh of snakes, whence the name Teriac or Theriac, from the snake " Tyrus." He consecrated this electuary to his royal protégé in a poem, enumerating all its ingredients, which Galen has preserved. This " Theriac " of Andromachus was introduced in all dispensatories, and was to be found in the Pharmacopœia Germanica of 1882 ; although the sixty-four ingredients given in the Dispensatory of Cordus, had dwindled to twelve. Theriac apparently occupied an important position in medicine down to the present century. Brunschwyck, in the beginning of the sixteenth century, writes : " When Theriac is to be made, each of its component parts should be exposed for at least two months in a public place, as at Venice, so that the wise men and doctors may inspect them, and determine whether or not they are fit for use."

Figure 70, from Brunschwyck's " Book for the Distillation of Composite Things," depicts a public display of vessels con-

* C. Plinius. Natural History, Vol. 25, Ch. 3.

taining the ingredients of Theriac.   The two human figures
represent a doctor and a druggist.   The two banners at the
corners of the table are decorated with Venetian lions, since
Venetian Theriac had the greatest reputation.   As the display
lasted several months, it certainly did not take place in the open
air, and the object of the illustration in placing the table on the
street, was to convey the idea that it was a public affair.   In

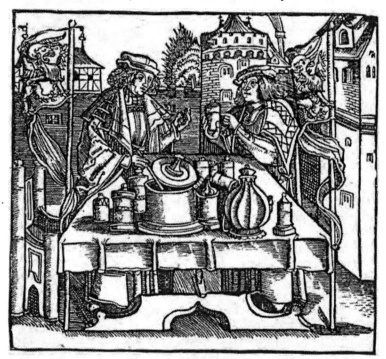

Fig. 70.

Germany, Theriac was prepared under official supervision ; the
Nuremburg apothecaries' ordinance provides that "no Theriac
shall in future be branded with the seal of the city unless it have
been previously examined and declared worthy of the same by
the doctors of medicine : every druggist must know the age of
the Theriac he sells.   Inasmuch as its action changes very
materially with age, the buyer should in all instances be informed
of this, so that he may not be deceived."   From the publicity

given the matter, the preparation of Theriac soon grew to be a state festival.   The last public preparation of Theriac took place at Nuremberg in 1754.   Since then it has gradually lost ground, and this Nestor of medicines now pines out its existence in out-of-the-way corners of a few antiquated pharmacies, where some spider has kindly spun a veil of mourning around it.   " Sic transit gloria mundi."   Even simples were obtained, according to the methods of Cordus, by very complicated procedures.   To prepare goat's-blood, formerly officinal, the druggist was obliged to feed a middle-aged buck, for one month, on celery, parsley and other Umbelliferæ, slaughter him in early summer when the sun was in the Tropic of Cancer, and dry the blood in an oven.

As the Dispensatory of Cordus was based entirely on the Galenico-Arabian school, the quinta essentia, tinctures, extracts and chemicals were wanting.   Distillation is briefly referred to in connection with a a few ethereal oils.   The distilled waters are omitted, not because they were not used, but because they were already so well known that, with the simples, they could be disregarded.   As the pharmacist had, in a great measure, to depend on foreign drugs, not always obtainable, because of defective methods of communication, he was tempted to practice substitution.   The custom of substitution advocated by Galen became so general in the Middle Ages that it was found expedient to designate the proper succedanea.   In an appendix to the Cordus Dispensatory, under the heading, " De Succedaneis Quid pro Quo," the Parisian physician enumerates the following substitutes :   " For the winter cherry, take common nightshade ; for colocynth, take castor beans ; for oil of laurel, take tar ; for storax, take castor ; for ginger, take pellitory root."   The substitutes do not always possess the same properties as the drugs that they supplant.   This custom probably had bad results.

In the 1592 edition of the Cordic Dispensatory edited by the Collegii Medici, American drugs are introduced, among them sarsaparilla and sassafras.   Oddly enough guaiac, which was administered to Ulric von Hutten, who died of syphilis, is not mentioned in this edition.   Another American drug was tobacco, used in skin diseases.   Among the chemicals are found the natural salts, alum, borax, saltpetre, etc. ; and a number of Sales arteficiosi.   These latter, sal absinthii, sal alkekengi, sal tartari, etc., are derived from the ash of plants and other substances, and consisted, in nearly every instance, of potash carbonate, while their name merely indicated the source whence they were derived. The artificial metallic salts, advocated by Paracelsus, are wanting in this edition. By the medical laws of 1592, attached to this Dispensatory, doctors and barbers are forbidden the use of the Paracelsian salts, such as Turpethum minerale, Mercurius præcipitatus, and Aurum vitæ.

A chapter on extracts and distilled waters was also incorporated. Plants and animals are pressed into service for this purpose. Aqua caponis and Aqua pullorum, "distillates of capon and pullet," are recommended as strengthening draughts and for inflammatory chest diseases. The 1598 edition of the Dispensatory, edited by the Collegii Medici, mentions among American drugs guaiac wood and white jalap (Radix mechoacannæ) now obsolete. To secure remedies from the animal kingdom the druggist was compelled to war with numerous animals ; he was called upon to furnish " Epar lupi," or Wolf-liver ; " Pulmo vulpis," fox lung. This still survives in the name of a syrup which contains no fox lung ; " Cervi os de corde," deer spine ; " Gallinarum stomachorum interiores pelliculæ," inner membrane of a chicken stomach, which still survives in " ingluvin ;" " Lana succida," sheep's wool ; " Lucii mandibula," the toothed jaw of a pike ; " Pili leporis " and "Talus leporis," rabbit hair and foot, still used by negroes ; " Græcum album," white excrement of a dog ; " Lapis fellus bovini," gallstones of an ox, still used in the shape of ox-gall ; swallows, sparrows, scorpions and centipedes were burned to ashes before being admitted into the kingdom of Æsculapius under the names of " Hirundines ustæ," " Passeres troglodytides," " Scorpiones," etc. Fat from every animal had to be procured. The sixteenth century pharmacist must have regarded with envious eye his plump fellow being, for he was also asked to keep in stock " poor sinner's fat," " Adeps hominis." " Cranium humanum," and " Oleum ossium humanorum " were also highly prized medicines. In this edition of the Dispensatary some of the more powerful metallic salts are introduced, such as white arsenic, the red and yellow arsenic sulphides, red precipitate, and corrosive sublimate. Of the mineral acids, sulphuric acid alone is mentioned. On the whole, the sixteenth century materia medica, as represented by the pharmacal body corporate, was comparatively refined. Cordus' Dispensatory contains comparatively few of the disgusting remedies in use in the seventeenth and eighteenth centuries, the mere suggestion of which shocks modern taste.

Many of the larger German cities introduced pharmacopœias of their own in the sixteenth century. Thus, in 1564, the "Pharmacopœia seu Medicamentarium pro Republica Augustana," was published at Augsburg, edited by the physician, Adolf Occo. In 1565 the Pharmacopœia of the City of Cologne was issued. A pharmacopœia was also published at Basel, by Dr. Foes, in the year 1561.

The sixteenth century was quite prolific in pharmacopœias. One was published at Mantua, Italy, in 1559, and one at Bergamo, in 1580. In Spain, the University town of Salamanca caught the spirit of the age by publishing a Pharmacopœia in 1588. These all bore some resemblance to the work of Cordus, which was but natural, since all bore traces of the Italian influence.

In the seventeenth century (1601), Spain, at the Great University of Salamanca, published the first new Pharmacopœia. In this century the influence of the separation of the apothecaries from the grocers in England, was shown in the necessity felt for some official standard, whence came the first English Pharmacopœia, the Pharmacopœia Londinensis, published in 1618. Subsequent editions of this work were published in 1650, 1677, 1721 and 1746. The early English pharmacopœias were largely compilations from the works of Mesuë, Nicolaus, and authors of this class, even as late as 1721.

The College of Physicians, in the preface to their 1746 edition of the Pharmacopœia, declare that "it is certainly a disgrace and just reproach if pharmacy should any longer abound with these inartificial and irregular mixtures, which the ignorance of the first ages introduced, and the perpetual fear and jealousies enforced ; against which the ancients endlessly busied themselves in the search of antidotes, which, for the most part, they superstitiously and dotingly derived from oracles, dreams and astrological fancies ; and, vainly hoping to frame compositions that might surely prevail against every species of poison, they amassed together whatever they had imagined to be endowed with alexipharmic powers. By this procedure the simplicity of physic was lost, and a wantonness in mixing, enlarging and accumulating took place, which has continued even to our own time." The Lyons Pharmacopœia long remained without a French competitor, for the first Pharmacopœia issued at Paris appeared in 1637. This was republished in 1639 as a Codex. Burdigal published its own Pharmacopœia in 1643 ; Toulons followed its example in 1648, and Valenciennes in 1651.

In the Netherlands, each of the prominent cities issued its own Pharmacopœia ; Amsterdam in 1636 ; Leyden in 1638 ; Brussels in 1639 ; Lille in 1640 ; Gand and The Hague in 1652 ; Utrecht and Louvaine in 1656 ; and Antwerp in 1661.

A pharmacopœia also appeared at Stralsund in 1645. The first Danish pharmacopœia, the " Pharmacopœia Hofmensis," was published in 1658.

In 1666, the fifth and last edition of the Cordic Dispensatory left the press. On the title-page of this edition is the copperprint reproduced on the first page of this chapter, Fig. 69. The lower part furnishes a birds-eye view of Nuremburg, while above and suspended in the clouds is seen a disciple of Æsculapius, mounted on a dragon, and directing four fiery steeds. Materia medica had undergone a great change since the preceding edition (1612) was issued. The list of remedies of animal origin was greatly augmented, and excrementitious substances were given special prominence. Medical cannibalism also increased in an alarming degree. Belts of human skin and woman butter enter upon the scene ; boy's urine, distilled with Hungarian vitriol, produced the Spiritus antipilepticus, an empyreumatic distillate employed in epilepsy. After the same formula Spiritus calvariæ humanæ and Spiritus ossium humanorum were prepared. Besides these disgusting remedies, whose adoption does not redound to the glory of medicine in the seventeenth century, many useful remedies were also introduced, which have retained their reputation to the present day. Cinchona is mentioned for the first time. Among American drugs still in use, Jalap, Peru and Tolu balsam are added. The tinctures and essences recommended by Paracelsus, and the number of

"Salia" and "Chymica," have also been multiplied. Ammonia carbonate, mixed with a variety of empyreumatic substances, comes in for its share of attention under the names of "Sal volatile cranii humani," "cornu cervi," "succini," "viperarum" and "urinæ." "Sal jovis" is prepared by dissolving zinc-ash, and "Sal saturni" by dissolving red lead in vinegar." "Mercurius præcipitatus albus" is prepared by dissolving mercury in nitric acid, and the adding to this a solution of sodium chloride. The resulting precipitate is a mild mercury chloride, identical with our white precipitate. Antimony, although not mentioned in this Dispensatory, had found a wide application in medicine. Antimony goblets were in use in the seventeenth century in convents. Monks addicted to wine were compelled to use these goblets. When the wine remained in contact with the metal for a brief period, it dissolved the antimony, forming a wine of antimony, which nauseated, and was said to have created an aversion to the favorite drink. The everlasting pills, "Pillulæ perpetuæ," of our forefathers, were also made of the metallic antimony. These were handed down from generation to generation as a precious heirloom, for, as a contemporaneous writer says: "Though they may have passed through the system an hundred times, they will always purge, and one will scarcely notice any diminution in their size."

In the 1666 edition of the Cordic Dispensatory so many chemicals, extracts and tinctures are mentioned, together with the old galenical formulas, that it may properly be called a representative work of the medical era foreshadowed by Paracelsus. With the exception of the alkaloids (not discovered until the nineteenth century) it contains all classes of remedies found in modern pharmacopœias. The first Swedish pharmacopœia, "The Pharmacopœia Holmensis," appeared in 1686.

The first Prussian pharmacal standard was the "Dispensatorum Brandenburgii," issued in 1698. Toward the close of the seventeenth century Spain published Pharmacopœias at Barcelona in 1686, and at Saragossa in 1698. The first Swiss Pharmacopœia, "The Pharmacopœia Helvetiorum," appeared in 1677. Haarlem, in Holland, issued a Pharmacopœia in 1693. The eighteenth century saw several new Pharmacopœias issued. The first Austrian Pharmacopœia was issued in 1739, and was revised by Störck in 1774. The first Bohemian Pharmacopœia appeared at Prague in 1739. Even Persia issued one in 1771, the "Makzan el Adwyn."

Dort, in Holland, issued one in 1708, and Almeria, in Spain, one in 1724.

In consequence of the efforts of Dr. Tilton, of Delaware, to reform the commissary department of Washington's Army, the first American Pharmacopœia was published at Philadelphia in 1778.

Not until the troubles of 1789 had quieted down did the first Irish Pharmacopœia appear in 1794.

As an illustration of the character of English Dispensatories in the eighteenth century the following formula is cited from the "Pharmacopœia Officinalis Extemporanea" or "Complete English Dispensatory," London, 1741.

Vinum Millepedum (*Hog-Lice Wine*).—Take hog-lice, half a pound, put them alive into two pounds of white port wine, and after some days' infusion strain and press out very hard; then put in saffron two drachms, salt of steel one drachm, and salt of amber two scruples, and after three or four days strain and filter for use. This is an admirable medicine against the jaundice, dropsy or any cachectic habit. It greatly deterges all the viscera, and throws off a great deal of superfluous humors by urine. It may be given twice a day, two ounces at a time.

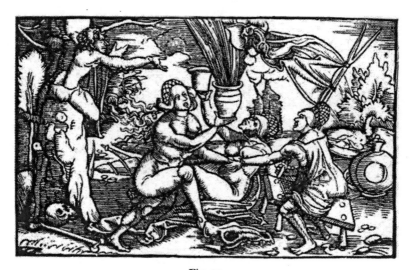

Fig. 71.
DEMONS OF DISEASE.
(From a book published A. D 1500).

" Now the magic fire prepare,
And from graves uprooted tear
Trees, whose horrors gloomy spread
Round the mansions of the dead ;
Bring the eggs and plumage foul
Of a midnight shrieking owl.
Be they well besmeared with blood
Of the blackest venom'd toad ;
From their various climates bring
Every herb that taints the spring ;
Then into the charm be thrown,
Snatch'd from famished bitch, a bone ;
Burn them all with magic flame
Kindled first by Colchian dame.''
                        —HORACE (Ode V, Book V).

Chapter Nine.

Medical Superstition.

UPERSTITION, the sponsor for miracle, and half-brother of faith, in the early centuries so dominated all fields of human endeavor, that it would be a difficult matter to name a science under whose cloak it has not practiced its wild pranks. The exact science of astronomy lay hidden in astrology, which reared a numerous progeny of augurs, soothsayers and interpreters of dreams. It was parent to the many simpletons who, misled by alchemy, endeavored, with the aid of the "philosopher's stone," to turn everything into gold, and make man immortal. Religious superstitions gave birth to sorcery, to apparitions, hobgoblins and phantoms; and prompted the interpreters of human laws to institute the abominable ordeals of fire and water, subsequently eclipsed in cruelty by the witchcraft laws. It is not astonishing that superstition should have usurped a seat and secured even legal recognition in the domain of medicine, when its fetichtic origin is remembered. The medical literature of the Middle Ages shows that many devotees of the art of healing exerted the ignoble skill of swimming with the tide of superstition, and of subordinating their profession to its mandates.

Medical superstition was largely based on certain views as to the nature of disease. Before man had accustomed himself to look for cause and effect in the domain of nature, and before physiology had cleared up the secrets of the mechanical processes associated with life, the cause of disease was sought for, not in the degenerative changes and perverted tissue metamorphosis of the body itself, but in the influence of some external evil agent, promptly personified, in accordance with the custom of early man, when he could find no other explanation for natural mutations affecting his well-being. A higher power, a demon under the guise of disease, took possession of its victim. This view of disease was not only almost universally accepted by the illiterate classes, but was so firmly rooted in the minds of learned physicians that traces of it are detectable in medical works of the eighteenth century. An eminent professor of Medical Jurisprudence in an American college, displayed decided traces of these old superstitions when, in October, 1888, he publicly stated that insanity of the sexual perversion type was an evidence of demoniacal possession. Certain outcast clergymen reap a golden harvest by pretending to exorcise the insane in the larger cities of the United States. With these facts in mind, it is not surprising that in the Middle Ages, mental diseases, epilepsy and nightmare were, without hesitation, declared to be due to visitations of ghosts and spirits.

Brunschwyck's "Book for Distilling Composite Things" has a chapter entitled "A Good Water to Drive out Demons and Demonic Spirits," which is introduced by a picture of a number of these diabolical monsters (Figure 71). When forced to contend with such conceptions, the efforts of the healing art were necessarily directed along different channels than at the present day, and consisted in great part of banishing and warding off the encroachments of these demons of disease. The most varied means were adopted to accomplish this end. Talismen and amulets were much in favor. These means of protection, still employed by some people, were formerly extensively prescribed by physicians. As late as 1731 the "Dispensatorium Regium Electorale Borusso-Brandenburgicum" contains a formula for an amulet to ward off the plague, the terror of the Middle Ages. This formula seems rather to have originated in a witch's-kitchen than in the august College of Physicians of the youthful Prussian kingdom. The following is the formula, from a Pharmacopœia one hundred and fifty years old :

"*Helmont's Amulet for the Plague.*—Although some may disparage the virtues of this remedy, it has nevertheless proven its efficacy in many instances, particularly during the war between the imperialists and rebels in Hungary, where the plague raged in a terrible manner. It gained such a reputation throughout the country that all 'barbers and blear-eyed witches' are already acquainted with its virtues. It is prepared in the following manner: Large, old frogs, caught in the month of June, are hung up by their hind legs over a dish covered with wax, which has been placed over a moderate fire. After a few days the frogs discharge horrible fumes and slaver, which attract every kind of worms and flies. These stick to the wax, and add their own drivel to the mess. When the frogs are dead, roast and mix them with the carefully preserved mixture of wax and drivel, and shape this compound into small rolls, or imitate the shapes of frogs. One of these is sewn into a cloth, and worn in the region of the heart, suspended by a silk thread around the neck. The longer one wears these the more certainly will he be protected from the ravages of the plague."

The "Corpus Pharmaceutico-Chymico-Medicum Universale," of Joh. H. Jünkens, published in 1697, contains a still richer collection of similar formulas. The supposition was, that disease entertained the same dislike for these disgusting and nauseating substances as the human being, and the wearer of them, therefore, had nothing to fear from the demons of disease. It is for this reason that the component parts of many amulets are not of very delicate nature. For epistaxis, Jünkens, in his " Universal Pharmacopœia," recommends the following compound under the euphonious name of "Sacculus pro amuleto in hæmorrhagia narium Senneri." "A small bag of red silk, filled with frog's ash, moss from a human skull, sea beans, frog's-root, etc., is worn suspended from the neck by a silken thread." The moss from human skull, "Usnea cranii humani," was either Parmelia saxatilis or Parmelia omphalodes. Lemery, in the "Cours de Chimie," published in 1675, says of it: "When the skulls have been exposed to the air for many years, a kind of green moss grows upon them which is called Usne. It is imported from Ireland, where it is customary to allow executed criminals to hang on posts in the field until they drop off piecemeal. After the skin and meat have disappeared, the moss develops on the skull. It is very astringent, and stops bleeding when applied externally. Taken internally it is also good for epilepsy, for it contains an abundance of volatile cranial salts."

Sea beans are the lids of a certain snail's shell (Turbo cochlus, rugosus, etc). The shells were worn as amulets for epistaxis, used as a vermifuge and diuretic, and applied to the abdomen in colic. Oswald Troll, in his "Basilica Chymica," gives minute directions for preparing amulets, as follows :

Zenexton seu Xenzethon Paracelsi.—First you have an instrument made for modeling tablettes that shall weigh 1½ drachms each. This instrument is to consist of three parts. (1) An upper plate engraved with a seal, embodying a snake. (2) A lower part made in the shape of an anvil, with a scorpion engraved on the upper surface ; and (3) a ring to retain the mass when it is compressed between the upper and lower pieces. The instrument should be made at a time when sun and moon enter the sign of the scorpion. The tablettes should also be made at this time, or, at least, when the moon enters the sign of the scorpion ; for in this manner the things on high and those of the lower regions are married by a sympathetic and inseparable union. These amulets or constellated tablettes are composed of

" 2 ounces dried frogs.
  Zenith juvencularum (Sanguinis menstrui primi), as much as you can secure.
  ½ ounce white or red arsenic.
  3 drachms tormentilla.
  1 drachm pearls (that have not been perforated).
  ½ drachm each of corals, hyacinths and emeralds.
  2 scruples of oriental saffron.
  To please the sense of smell, a few grains of musk or ambergris may be added.
    All parts are now finely powdered and made into a mass by the admixture
    of tragacanth and rosewater."

The tablettes (Pentacula) are now formed at the time mentioned, and by the instrument described above ; or, if one prefer, they may be made in the shape of a heart.

"*Use.*—These Pentacula are worn between the wearing apparel in the region of the heart. They not only fortify the wearer against the plague, but also counteract all poisons and nullify pernicious astral influences."

Precious stones were reputed to have power to protect from disease, and were consequently worn for this purpose, set in gold, silver or steel. Diamonds worn on the left arm were a protection against madness, wild animals, war, quarrels, poison and delirium. That precious stones were quite generally pressed into this service, is witnessed by the "Zenexton pro ditioribus Magnatibus," the preparation of which is thus described by Oswald Troll :

"A capsule of purest gold is made, and into it a golden tube, whose walls are perforated by numerous openings, is securely fastened. On one side of the capsule a brilliant sapphire is attached, and surrounded by four frog-stones; the other side being similarly embellished by a large hyacinth. The capsule is then filled with ground frogs and the best of vinegar, and the perforated tube running through the centre of the capsule is filled with shreds of linen, 'Quod primo virginis menstruo, quæ annum decimum quintum nondum excesserit madefacum fuit,' having a care that the contents of the capsule and those of the tube may come in contact by way of the openings in the latter. This mutual contact is productive of an element of sympathy, which in its turn is antagonistic to all poisons, as has been conclusively proven by those who have worn this amulet during epidemics of plague."

Incantations were used to drive out disease. The peasantry in many parts of Europe place more confidence to-day in the conjuring and appeasing of disease by magical agencies than in the practices of qualified physicians. These ceremonies are ordinarily directed by pock-marked, wrinkled, blear-eyed old women. After repeating some traditional mystic rite, which, on account of its mere verbal transmission, varies greatly, the Holy Trinity is invoked, and fire drawn from a stone, by means of a steel, three times in succession. The sick person leaves the old hag inspired with new hope, and, since time cures many ills, the faith in these village sibyls will not soon die out.

Healing powers were attributed not only to spoken but written words. The words chosen for this purpose were usually entirely meaningless, or taken from some oriental language. For the less he comprehends their meaning the more is the patient convinced of their deep magical significance. Where the modern physician prescribes quinine for fever, his ancient predecessors prescribed the simple word "Abracadabra," written on a piece of paper, which was swallowed by the patient, whereupon the fever was expected to leave the body. Small triangular slips of paper, upon which words from the Bible were written by consecrated hands, were taken by women in difficult confinements. The belief was current that the executioner, as the servant of death, could issue passports for the latter, which would protect the bearer from the hangman, from death and wounds.   The use of these passports with them still prevailed among the soldiery of the Thirty-years War.   The methods and notions involved in the preparation of amulets demonstrate what a powerful factor astrology was at one time in medicine.

The custom of casting the patient's horoscope was almost universal during the Middle Ages.   On the notion of a relationship between the metals and the planets, elsewhere described, a metal was frequently chosen as a remedy, which bore the same name as the planet which most frequently entered the constellation associated with the patient's being.   At the present day, even, many people will take a vermifuge only at the waning of the moon.   A foreboding appears to have permeated the notions entertained in the Middle Ages, that the individual members of creation held a certain mutual relationship to each other ; no attempt was made to explain this interdependence by natural laws, but the belief was accepted of a magical bond which united all creation, and of a secret sympathy permeating all nature.

The preponderating notion that the world was created for the exclusive benefit of man, conditioned an affinity between the entire cosmos and the microcosm, and led to the belief that the relationship existing between certain objects in nature and man, could be detected either by outward similarities or by secret signs and agencies.   Such notions led medicine into strange channels.   Remedies were consequently not administered on the principle of their action, but because of their supposed sympathetic relationship to the patient or his disease.   Liverwort (Hepatica triloba) was used in liver disease, because its leaves had the shape of that organ, and on the brown under-surface its color.   Viper's bugloss (Echium vulgare), whose flower simulates a snake's head, was of course good for snake-bite.   Celandine (Chelidonium majus) was looked upon as a present from heaven (cœli donum), since its yellow flower and yellow sap were conclusive evidence that it was presented to man by the Creator to cure jaundice.   Ramson (Gladiolus communis) has sword-like leaves, and its bulbs, covered with a net-like skin, resemble the meshes of an armor, all of which demonstrated that Providence had designed this plant to render man proof against the accidents of the battlefield ; hence the old knights frequently carried one of these roots under their steel armor, believing that they were thereby not only protected against wounds, but were ensured a victory.

At the present day roots and herbs are still used in connection with superstitious practices. Many a peasant in the Black Forest, at Christmas-time, buys a root each of Radix victorialis longa and Radix victorialis rotunda, and buries this pair under the door-sill, hoping thereby to banish all witches and demons of disease, which are prone to wander about, particularly on Christmas eve.

The peasant of the Hartz mountains has not heard of the modern scape-goats, the "bacteria." When his milk turns blue, he charges this to witches. To protect his milk from them nothing, in his opinion, is so effective as the blue-eyed ground ivy (Glechoma hederacea). He winds a wreath of it, and on the Maynight " Walpurgis' night," when the witches from all quarters of the globe hold high carnival on the Brocken, he milks his cows through this wreath so that his milk shall be protected for the coming year.

It was considered an easy matter to transfer a disease to anything with which it had a secret sympathy (an interchangeable term for affinity and relationship). The action of the so-called mummy or sympathetic egg, extensively employed by Theophrastus Bombastus Paracelsus, of Hohenheim, in the sixteenth century, and by his followers, the so-called Paracelsists, after him, was accounted for on this notion. To prepare this mummy an empty chicken's egg, filled with warm blood from a healthy individual, was carefully sealed and at once placed under a brooding hen, so that its vitality should not escape with the decreasing temperature. After a few weeks it was placed in an oven and subjected to heat for a length of time sufficient to bake bread. An egg prepared in this manner was supposed to cure every disease ; for, as the blood was supposed to be the true seat of disease, every disease would naturally have a greater affinity for this egg which contained blood in such a concentrated form. The disease being thus bound to escape to the sympathetic egg, it was only necessary, for a cure in a given case, to place the egg in contact with the diseased part and subsequently bury it in the earth.

Trees were supposed to be effective mediums to charm away disease. Since Judas was believed to have hanged himself to an elder tree, the elder was supposed to possess magical powers. Inasmuch as the administration of an infusion of its leaves causes diaphoresis and heat, the tea was, on the principle of "Similia similibus curantur," credited with being in secret sympathy with fevers, and would cure them if begged to do so in a suppliant mood. For this reason, at the present day, fever patients in North Germany repair to the elder tree, and speak these words:

> "O beloved elder tree,
> Of my fever set me free;
> Since Judas false from you did hang,
> I give to you my fev'rish pang."

The patient then breaks a twig from the tree and plants it in the ground, whereupon, if the cure progresses as it should, the fever leaves the sufferer and follows the course of the twig into the earth, like lightning gliding along the rod.

The price of the drug, also, is oftentimes of importance. In north Germany seven, and in France nine, are preferred numbers. When a sibyl buys camphor to wear in a bag for her rheumatism, she always buys nine-pence worth, as otherwise it would not help. The belief was current that certain remedies could cure a patient in absentia. One celebrated remedy of this kind was the wonderful weapon salve of Paracelsus, which consisted of boar's and bear's fat, rain-worms, hog's-brain, yellow sandal, mummy, bloodstone and moss from the skull of a hanged criminal, which latter was to be gathered at the waxing of the moon. The author of the formula says: "The virtues of this salve are remarkable, for with it you can heal all kinds of wounds, though the patient be miles away, provided you can but secure the weapon with which the wound was inflicted. This weapon must be greased once a day with this salve, then tied up in a clean linen cloth and preserved in a warm locality. It should be protected from dust and cold draughts, otherwise the patient would experience great pain and become delirious. Although this cure may appear supernatural, and consequently be discountenanced by many, I can, nevertheless, assure the reader that this is not the case, for those initiated in the natural sciences know from experience, and have proven by diligent research, that the cure is accomplished by means of a certain magnetic force that emanates from the stars, and acts upon the salve, conveying the latter's magnetic force through the air and to the wound."

The influence exerted by astrology on medicine in those days is again illustrated here. In Hesse, also, according to popular belief, patients were cured *in absentia*. In the case of a fractured limb, particularly of an animal, the surgical magician bandaged the broken leg of a table or chair, at the same time repeating his magic rite. The bandaged object was not to be interfered with for nine days, when at the expiration of this time, not the broken table-leg, but the patient's limb, would have re-united.

At all times man's most fervent desire has been to lift the veil that hides from him the future. Hieronymus Bock, in his "New Herb-Book of the Actions and Names of Herbs that Grow in Germany," Strassburg, 1551, relates that the large gall-nuts possess the property of disclosing whether the coming year will be a prosperous one, or whether war will desolate or pestilence rule the land. "In the month of January take a well-preserved gall-nut, and, on breaking it in two, you will find one of three things, a fly, a maggot, or a spider. The fly denotes war; the maggot, hard times; and the spider, disease." The vegetable excrescence known as the gall-nut is produced by the deposit of the eggs of the insect (Cynips gallæ tinctoria) in the bark and leaves of the oak (Quercus infectoria). This causes an increased flow of sap to these parts, and by the time the larvæ have fairly developed, they find themselves thoroughly protected by a pulpy growth. In the course of its generative metamorphosis the larva changes into a chrysalis, and finally into the gall insect, which escapes from the gall-nut. As the gall-insect failed to protect its discovery of the process of manufacturing gall-nuts, other insects, some of them resembling a spider more than a fly, encroach upon its prerogatives. This latter fact, coupled with the different stages of development in which the gall-insect is found during its generative changes, accounts for the various specimens of animal life met with in the gall-nut.

The healing art of old was also called upon to prop up the

memory. One remedy of this kind is the fruit of Anacardium. "One-half ounce of this taken internally strengthens the intellect, banishes forgetfulness, and is good for weakness of the brain resulting from cold or moisture." Many of these superstitions still persist to the present day. The "hoodoo" and the "mascot" play an active part in modern life. Witchcraft trials, under a modified form, have recently occurred in a western State; and the "witch doctress" is in use in Brooklyn. The old fetichtic ideas hold their own. With respectable American college professors proclaiming their belief in demon possession; with medical journals containing articles advocating similar doctrines; with Georgia medical dreamers advocating "hairless dogs" in the treatment of rheumatism on the "sympathy" principle; with the "hunchback"-touching guard against disease in full luxuriance in an Atlantic city; with vast industries devoted to the manufacture of "patent" medicines, and a popular press teeming with their marvelous virtues, it is hardly time to boast about general enlightenment, and acridly criticise the Middle Ages. An age which accepts remedies prescribed by "spirits," "angels," etc., cannot be too tolerant of the errors of preceding periods.

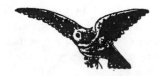

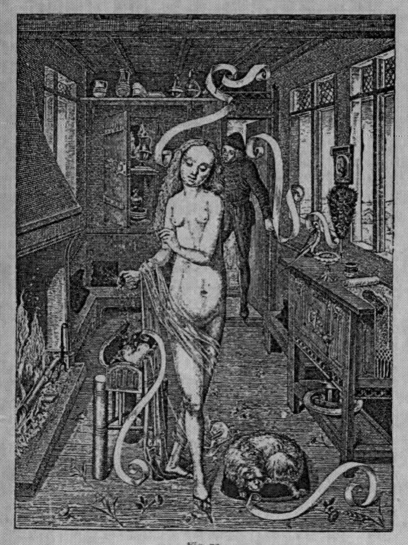

Fig. 72.

(137)

" Thou'lt find, this drink thy blood compelling,
Each woman beautiful as Helen."

—FAUST.

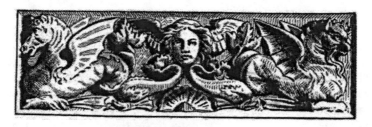

Chapter Ten.

Pharmacy and Magic of Love.

E important part which "love" plays in the drama of life, prepares us for the discovery that men and women, at a very early period, resorted to magical influences for exciting the affections. The belief existed among the older nations, as among the lower orders to-day, that there were magical and physical agents by means of which one person could secure the passionate love of another. The belief in the magical agents was a survival of the teachings of fetichism. The belief in the physical agents arose from the influence certain drugs were observed to exert on the mind. From the "wine which maketh glad the heart of man," to the "grief dispelling nepenthe" of Homer, was but a step. Nepenthe was presented by Helen to Telemachus at the house of Menelaus the Good, that he might forget his sorrows. The formula for this drink had been obtained from "Polydamnoes, wife of Thous of Egypt, where the rich earth brings forth precious but also many dangerous herbs." The composition of Homer's "nepenthe" cannot now be determined, but it seems certain that the "nepenthes destillatoria" of Linnæus was not its source. It has been asserted that it was prepared from the Egyptian henbane (hyoscyamus datura and albus) used by the priests to appease the evil principle. Typhon Miquel* declares that the poppy, whose properties were known before the days of Hippocrates, corresponds most to the description given of νηπενθες. It has been said that it was a decoction of Indian Hemp, whose intoxicating properties were known from a very remote period.

* Homeric Flora. (139)

Herodotus, "Father of History," says that the "Scythians place in the ground three stakes inclining toward each other, and fasten woolen blankets tightly over them. In the space between the stakes is a pan filled with red-hot stones. There grows in their country a species of hemp which resembles flax, only it is taller and thicker. The Scythians throw the seeds of this hemp upon the hot stones, when immediately a thick vapor arises, more dense than in a Grecian sweat-bath. This steaming takes the place of a bath with the Scythians, and under its influence they give utterance to shouts of delight." Hasheesh is still extracted from gunjah, the leaves, flowers and fruits of the female hemp plant. This, in Mohammedan countries, takes the place of alcoholic drinks, and was used by the "Old Man of the Mountain" to transport his dupes to an imaginary paradise filled with houris. In moderate doses it produces cheerfulness, and hence has been used in the treatment of melancholia. The Asiatics call it the "Exciter of Desire," the "Cementer of Friendship" and the "Laugh Provoker." "Bang," used by the Malays as an intoxicant, contains hasheesh. As hasheesh, bang and opium (when smoked) produce voluptuous visions and sensations, the conclusion was naturally drawn that these or similar agents could produce love. The older fetichism also gave rise to the belief in the love charm. From the two conceptions sprang the Greek myth Circe. The traffic in charms was not so dangerous as that in philters, which were an early source of revenue to the Greeks. The results of this traffic were so infamous that it was forbidden by Lycurgus and Solon, whose laws crushed out the native dealers. Later, foreign sorceresses gained a foothold on Grecian soil. Keramiekos, "the Potters' Quarter" of Athens, where laborers and tradespeople dwelt, swarmed with Phrygian and Thessalian hags who sold poisons, aphrodisiacs and love-charms. The majority of these substances were no doubt narcotics.

In ancient times the mandrake (Mandragora officinalis), which grows very abundantly in Greece, enjoyed the greatest reputation as a philter. For ages it had been reputed to have magical properties. It is probably referred to by Homer when speaking of the excellent remedy that Hermes gave to Odysseus to counteract the charmed draught administered by Circe; "Black is its root, and milk-white its flower, Moly 'tis named by

the gods ; For mortals 'tis difficult to dig it, but to celestials all
is possible." The black, carrot-like root, which in its lower half
frequently parts into two branches, and is beset by small hirsute
filaments, somewhat resembles the human form, whence the
name given by Pythagoras, $\alpha \nu \vartheta \rho \omega \pi o \mu \acute{o} \rho \varphi \eta$—man-like shape.
Columella called it the " Planta semihominis " — half-man plant.

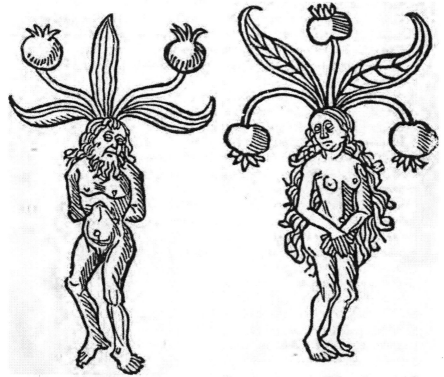

alraun man cclvii Calraun fraw cclvii c

Fig. 73.

MALE MANDRAKE.

Fig. 74.

FEMALE MANDRAKE.

Pliny the Elder says that " overindulgence in it will cause death,
but in moderation it produces a gentle soporific effect. An infusion of it is taken for snake-bite, and is given before operations
to dull the senses, for in some instances the mere smelling of it
will induce sleep." Frontinus says that Marhabel, when sent by

the Carthaginians to subdue the rebellious Africans, used this soporific quality of mandrake to vanquish the enemy. He placed mandrake in wine, and feigning a retreat, allowed this to fall into the hands of the enemy who, drinking, fell into deep slumber and were easily captured.

Dioscorides, Pliny, and later botanists, differentiate between male and female plants, probably varieties of the same species. Dioscorides calls the male " Morion," and the female, " Thridacias." The "Ortus sanitatis," of 1486, has figures of two mandrakes reproduced in figures 73 and 74.

The artist enormously exaggerated the natural appearance of the roots.

The King James version of the Bible says that Reuben gathered mandrake, and his mother, Leah, bribed Rachel,* the favorite, with them, to permit her to enjoy Jacob's affection.

The old chap books turned the biblical story into the use of mandrake root, as a philter, by Leah. It therefore gained great repute as a love potion in the period antecedent to the "Reformation." Theriac dealers and hunters carved the roots into shapes resembling little men and women, and often substituted the root of Bryonia. They then sunk grass and millet-seeds into the head part, and buried these in moist ground until filaments grew which resembled hair. When dried, these figures were called mandrakes, and were bought at a high price for household deities. In secret they were richly dressed, received a share of each meal, and were bathed in wine on Saturday evening. They,

Fig. 75.
MANDRAKE.

like "fern-seed," had the power to confer invisibility. They made the poor rich, healed all diseases, and made their owner fortunate in love.

Figure 75 represents one of these mandrakes now in the Germanic Museum at Nuremburg.

The price of the root was enhanced by the story that it grew under the gallows of a victim of a judicial murder, and could

* Genesis xxx, 14-16.

only be dug at great risk to life, since that its horrible shrieks, when drawn from the earth, might strike the hearer dead. In gathering it the ears had to be closed with wax. One end of a rope was tied to the root, and the other to a black dog, who perished in pulling it out. Figure 76 (a reduced copy of a fifteenth century picture, in the Germanic Museum), represents this procedure.

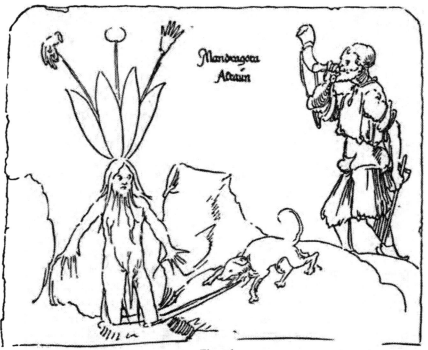

Fig. 76.

As an additional precaution, the digger blows a horn to drown the death-dealing shrieks of the mandrake. Goethe, on one occasion refers to this tradition :

> " One twaddles and rants about the black dog,
> Another prates and dotes on the mandrake."

Even Pliny speaks of the dangers associated with the digging of the mandrake. "Whoever would dig it must avoid having the wind against him, and when he digs should face in the direction of the setting sun."

Another love charm employed by the Greeks was the Thessalian herb "Catananche," which cannot now be identified. The modern "Catananche cœrulea" is identical with the "Datisca cannabina" of Dioscorides. Pliny mentions Catananche very briefly, as follows: "For the purpose of exposing this humbug, it suffices to say, that the only reason that this plant was supposed to possess powers to charm, was because that, upon drying, it assumed a shape somewhat resembling the talons of a hawk." On the basis of this meagre report, some feel justified in declaring it to be "Ornithopus compressus," or the Astragalus pugniformis. Properties similar to those of Catananche were ascribed to the plant "Cemos," probably the Plantago cretica.

When these physical agents did not produce the desired result, or when they produced grave mischief, incantations were employed to secure the love so much coveted. Theocritus, who lived at Syracuse 300 B. C., vividly describes these incantations in his "Sorceress." The enamored Simaetha, a maid of Syracuse, finding herself betrayed and slighted by her beloved Delphis, determines upon regaining his love by charms and incantations. For this purpose she repairs with her servant, Thestylis, by the light of the moon, to the cross-roads between the city and the sea. The object of their incantations is to cause the person, on whom the charm is designed to work, to suffer like the inanimate objects used in the ceremonial. She begins the rite by encircling the cauldron with bands of finest wool. She then calls upon the gentle Selene, and the repulsive Hecate (whom Theocritus identifies with Artemis), to assist her. Hecate, thought to be a three-headed, snake-haired and snake-footed witch of extraordinary size, disguised in black, and accompanied by giant dogs, wandered about at midnight, and as she loitered about the cross-roads was called the cross-roads goddess. At the beginning of the incantation proper, Simaetha spins a top, and during the incantation, whilst sacrificing the necessary objects, she speaks the following words, in which she discloses all the varied emotions of a rejected lover :

" Where are my laurels? and my philters, where ?
Quick bring them, Thestylis—the charm prepare;
This purple fillet round the cauldron strain,
That I with spells may prove my perjur'd swain ;
For since he rapt my door twelve days are fled,
Nor knows he whether I'm alive or dead ;
Perhaps to some new face his heart's inclined,
For love has wings, and he a changeful mind.
To the Palæstra with the morn I'll go,
And see and ask him, why he shuns me so ?
Meanwhile my charms shall work : O queen of night !
Pale moon, assist me with refulgent light ;
My imprecations I address to thee,
Great goddess, and infernal Hecatè
Stain'd with black gore, whom even gaunt mastiffs dread,
Whene'er she haunts the mansions of the dead ;
Hail, horrid Hecatè ! and aid me still
With Circe's power, or Perimeda's skill,
Or mad Medea's art,—Restore, my charms,
My lingering Delphis to my longing arms."

" The cake's consum'd—burn, Thestylis, the rest
In flames ; what frenzy has your mind possest ?
Am I your scorn, that thus you disobey,
Base maid, my strict commands ?—Strew salt and say,
' Thus Delphis' bones I strew,—Restore, my charms,
The perjur'd Delphis to my longing arms.' "

" Delphis inflames my bosom with desire ;
For him I burn this laurel in the fire ;
And as it fumes and crackles in the blaze,
And without ashes instantly decays,
So may the flesh of Delphis burn,—My charms,
Restore the perjur'd Delphis to my arms.

" As melts this waxen form, by fire defac'd,
So in love's flames may Myndian Delphis waste ;
And as this brazen wheel, tho' quick roll'd round,
Returns, and in its orbit still is found,
So may his love return,—Restore my charms,
The lingering Delphis to my longing arms.

" I'll stew the bran, Diana's power can bow
Rough Rhadamanth, and all that's stern below,
Hark ! hark ! The village dogs ! the goddess soon
Will come—the dogs terrific bay the moon—
Strike, strike the sounding brass,—Restore, my charms,
Restore false Delphis to my longing arms.

" Calm is the ocean, silent is the wind,
    But grief's black tempest rages in my mind,
    I burn for him whose perfidy betray'd
    My innocence ; and me, ah, thoughtless maid !
    Robb'd of my richest gem,—Restore, my charms,
    False Delphis to my long-deluded arms.

" I pour libations thrice, and thrice I pray ;
    O shine, great goddess, with auspicious ray .
    Whoe'er she be, blest nymph ! that now detains
    My fugitive in Love's delightful chains ;
    Be she forever in oblivion lost,
    Like Ariadne, 'lorn on Dia's coast,
    Abandon'd by false Theseus,—O, my charms,
    Restore the lovely Delphis to my arms.

" Hippomanes, a plant Arcadia bears,
    Makes the colts mad, and stimulates the mares,
    O'er hills, thro' streams they rage ; O, could I see
    Young Delphis thus run madding after me,
    And quit the fam'd Palæstra ! O, my charms,
    Restore false Delphis to my longing arms.

" This garment's fringe, which Delphis wont to wear,
    To burn in flames I into tatters tear.
    Oh, cruel Love ! that my best life-blood drains
    From my pale limbs, and empties all my veins,
    As leeches suck young steeds,—Restore, my charms,
    My lingering Delphis to my longing arms.

" A lizard bruis'd shall make a potent bowl,
    And charm, to-morrow, his obdurate soul ;
    Meanwhile this potion on his threshold spill,
    Where, though despis'd, my soul inhabits still ;
    No kindness he nor pity will repay ;
    Spit on the threshold, Thestylis, and say,
    ' Thus Delphis' bones I strew ',—Restore, my charms,
    The dear, deluding Delphis to my arms.
                    —FAWKE'S THEOCRITUS,
                          (Idyllum II, Pharmaceutica). "

Lucian, the satirist, who lived three hundred years after Theocritus, describes a love incantation in a dialogue between Melitta and Bacchis :

"*Bacchis*—There is, dear friend, an able sorceress in Syria. Her methods, Melitta, are simple ; she takes but a drachma and a loaf of bread, and upon this seven obolus must also lie, some salt, sulphur and a torch. These she takes, and a jug of wine is procured, and, if possible, a piece of clothing or the slippers "—

"*Melitta*—I have his slippers !"

"*Bacchis*—These she hangs from a nail, and under them burns the sulphur, and of the salt she also throws some into the fire. During this act she speaks the names of both parties, yours and his. Then she draws a top from her bosom and spins it, whilst, with fluent tongue, she repeats a magic rite in barbarous and dreadful sounding words. This is the way in which she did it that time, and shortly thereafter Phanias, in spite of his comrades' jeers and the entreaties of Phoebe, with whom he was together, returned to my arms, evidently in consequence of this incantation."

The Greeks used aphrodisiac preparations, which were termed Satyrion, from the satyrs, the symbols of sensuality. These satyrions were often composed of orchids, chosen on account of the suggestive shape of their bulbs. They were often destitute of aught but imaginary aphrodisiac properties. Pliny says that their properties often became manifest when taken into the hand, but were much more powerfully developed when taken in dry wines. Dogwort (Anacamptis pyramidalis), which has two bulbs, one withered and the other fresh and juicy, is called cynosorchis by Theophrastus, who says that in Thessaly the men drink the larger fresh root in goat's-milk as an aphrodisiac, and the smaller as a sexual sedative. They are therefore antagonistic. This belief in the aphrodisiac powers of the orchid was almost universal, and survives to-day in the popular designation of the bulb-pair, in some parts of the United States, as "Adam and Eve." Among the Northern nations the legend was prevalent that the giantess, Brana, presented Bronn-grass to her love, Halfdan, while Freya (the goddess of love), presented Freya-grass to those she met. Both "grasses" were orchids. The plant Cratægis was also used in satyrion. Of it two varieties were mentioned, "Thelygonos," the girl-producing, and "Androgonos," the boy-producing kind. They are supposed to be identical with the mercury-weed (Mercurialis tomentosa), which belongs to the Diœcia.

The superstitions associated with these bulbs no doubt sprung from their peculiar shape, for, in antiquity, the action of the drugs was supposed to depend on similarities and secret signs. Pliny further mentions, as ingredients of love-charms, the "Stergethron" (Sempervivium tectorum), "Horminos agrios" (Salvia silvestris," and the "sea-fennel" (Crithmum maritimum), which latter Hecate served to Theseus at table as a vegetable.

The practice of love-magic by the Egyptians is evident from numerous formulæ on the papyri unearthed by Ebers, who, in his "Uarda," gives an exquisite picture of an old sorceress Hekt. Paaker, the villain of the story, enters her cave to secure a love-charm. "At the side of the sorceress was a wheel suspended between the teeth of a wooden fork, and kept in perpetual motion. A large coal-black tom-cat cowered at her side, and sniffed at the heads of crows and owls deprived of their eyes. When Paaker entered the cave, the old crone shrieked : 'Does the water boil ? Then throw in the ape's eye and the ibis feather, and the linen rags with the black signs. * * * This alone binds hearts. Three is the man ; Four is the woman ; and Seven the indivisible ! ' "

The grammarian, Apion, of Oasis, in Egypt, who lived during the reign of the Emperors Tiberius and Claudius, maintains, according to Pliny, that the mere touching the herb Anacampseros (Sedum anacampseros), would rekindle love, even should hate have usurped its place.

At no time was there more barefaced deception practiced with oracles, spirits and conjurations ; never was the trade of the juggler and sorceress easier or more lucrative, and nowhere was the art of preparing love-charms better developed, than at Rome during the reign of the first emperors. The riches garnered in this capital of the world lent an air of ease to life, which led to all sorts of demoralizing practices.

Attempts were often made to exchange, by magical or medicinal means, these riches for the love so much courted and coveted by mankind in all ages. In this, the Sagæ and Medicæ willingly lent a helping hand. These closely allied Sagæ and Medicæ came from the ranks of immoral crones, who not only plied a lucrative trade in love-charms but treated venereal diseases, practiced abortion, and in cold blood suffocated burdensome newly-born infants in the folds of their dress. In the vile dens of these unprincipled women, the deadly Halicacabum, prepared from the winter cherry (Physalis somnifera) and the common night-shade (Solanum nigrum), was kept on sale for the removal of inconvenient rivals.

In reviewing the various Trychnos or Strychnos species, Pliny states that the Halicacabum, "in the dose of one drachm, awakens carnal desires, and causes visionary forms and pictures to appear as real. Double this dose will cause actual madness, and a further increase, death." At night the Sagæ culled poisonous herbs, and took bones and hair from the dead with which to prepare the vile decoctions used by them.

Horace, who one night met the notorious Canidia (mentioned by several Roman writers) on the Æsquilian Hill, the "Potter's Field" of Rome, thus describes her practices :

> " But oh ! nor thief, nor savage beast,
> That used these gardens to infest,
> E'er gave me half such care and pains
> As they, who turn poor people's brains
> With venom'd drug and magic lay—
> These I can never fright away.
> For when the beauteous queen of night
> Uplifts her head adorn'd with light,
> Hither they come, pernicious crones !
> To gather poisonous herbs and bones.
> Canidia, with dishevelled hair,
> (Black was her robe, her feet were bare),
> With Sagana, infernal dame !
> Her elder sister, hither came.
> With yellings dire they fill'd the place,
> And hideous pale was either's face.
> Soon with their nails they scrap'd the ground,
> And filled a magic trench profound
> With a black lamb's thick streaming gore,
> Whose members with their teeth they tore,
> That they may charm some sprite to tell
> Some curious anecdote from hell.
> The beldams then two figures brought ;
> Of wool and wax the forms were wrought ;
> The woolen was erect and tall,
> And scourg'd the waxen image small,
> Which in a suppliant, servile mood,
> With dying air just gasping stood.
> On Hecate one beldam calls ;
> The other to the furies bawls,
> While serpents crawl along the ground,
> And hell-born bitches howl around.
> The blushing moon, to shun the sight,
> Behind a tomb withdrew her light."
>
> —FRANCIS' HORACE (Satire VII).

One of Canidia's decoctions was known as the "cup of desire," but the ingredients of this draught have not been preserved.

According to the tradition, the most common ingredient of Roman philters was the "Hippomane." This, Pliny states, was said to possess such powers, that a brazen mare, in the casting of which Hippomane had been incorporated, caused stallions brought in its vicinity to be transported with passion. The old writers differ much as to the nature and origin of this drug. At all events it should not be confounded with the mancinella tree (Hippomane Mancinella), whose shade, as the legend says, will cause the death of the person sleeping in it. According to Theocritus it was an Arcadian herb, on eating which the horses became frantic. Pliny, however, says: "On the forehead of a new-born colt is found a fleshy protuberance, which is swallowed by the mother before allowing the colt to suckle. This fleshy growth was used by the Sagæ in the preparation of Hippomane." Ovid and Juvenal adopt this view of the nature of Hippomane. This matter admits of a very simple explanation. The colts, like the young of most animals, when born, are surrounded by a membrane. To facilitate the liberation of the colt, the mother swallows this and the afterbirth.* During this process a liquid, frequently mixed with a dark, solid mass, escapes, which latter was collected and, in all probability, was used in the preparation of the drug. Evidently Hippomane was already in part classed with the "Aphrodisiaca" which the Sagæ prepared, and which had actual aphrodisiac properties.

Satyrion is mentioned in the "Satyricon" of Petronius, which was written to satirize Nero. From the description there given, this potion seems to have been a very active aphrodisiac. As a rule, these drinks were known as "Aquæ amatrices," and were very much in vogue among the Romans. Substances of the most varied origin were incorporated in these infernal decoctions. Gall of wild boars, ambergris, turtle-eggs, sea-mullets, cuttlefish (the latter were known as "Uvæ marinæ"), smelts, cantharides, crickets and other animals and their products, were extracted by wine. The plant-kingdom contributed its share to these compounds. According to Martial, puff-balls, probably Lyco-

* Except in England.

perdon cervinum, and other fungi, were also employed. Ovid mentions a number of these substances, all of which were more or less injurious, and had many victims. Lucretius, who, in his didactic poem, " De Rerum Natura," advocated the philosophy of Epicurus, is said to have taken his life during the delirium of a terrible satyriasis caused by these draughts. Lucullus, the bon vivant, came to his end in a similar manner. His freedman, Kalisthenes, gave him a love-drink for the purpose of retaining his good-will forever, from the effects of which he died.*

In the Middle Ages, the belief in philters was wide-spread. Gottfried, of Strassburg, in the thirteenth century, states that the love of " Tristan and Isolde," was the result of a love-drink. The mother prepared a love-draught, which Isolde, her daughter, princess of Eyreland, was to drink with her betrothed, King Mark, upon reaching Cornwall. By a servant's oversight, the potion is divided between Tristan and Isolde, and no sooner had they tasted of it, when both fell deeply in love. Although the author of " Tristan and Isolde," is very frank, and describes lovers in attitudes which modern erotic poets pass over in silence, he does not disclose the ingredients of this draught.

In Germany, henbane (Hyoscyamus niger) enjoyed considerable reputation as a philter. It was the root of this plant which the rat-catcher of Hamelin employed to secure a kiss from Regina, the proud daughter of the Burgomaster Gruwelholt. The sequel of this beautiful romance reveals that during the celebration of her engagement to Heribert, her love for the rat-catcher broke out ; and

> " She flew to the arms of the fiddler,
> And love distracted, caressed him."

In " The Book of Nature " of Megenberg, written in 1350, various herbs are recommended as philters. " The vervain (Verbena officinalis), which creates love between man and woman, is of great service to sorcerers ; and this they know full well that have been in the net, but they will not let the secret out." Vervain, in Anglo-Saxon countries, hindered " witches of their will."

Love-charms begin now to assume a purely fetichtic char-

* Plutarch, chapter 45.

acter. The influence of Christianity turned the inspired sorceress of pagan days into witches. The Nicors of the Northern races became united into " Old Nick." The god " Pan " of the Romans became the Devil. The superstitions of the people did not vanish but became changed. Rites which had been divine became devilish. The hysterical females and nervous men who had been the admired of the gods and goddesses, became the devil's brides or husbands, the incubi and succubi of the Middle Ages. The witches of the period, like the fortune tellers of the present day, sought to inspire terror in order to secure power. The older superstitions descended to them from the traditional practices of the pagan sorceress, but became degraded into the older fetichtic ideas of the soul of the individual entering into his or her belongings, whence their advocacy and administration of so many disgusting agents for awakening love. They advised the lover to secure such things from the adored one as would be likely to possess the peculiarities of the individual in the highest degree. The hair, nails and pieces of soiled linen were exceedingly valued, and were burned to ashes and thus administered as love powders. Females frequently sent their chosen ones the co-called " love-cakes," promising themselves great results therefrom. To prepare these the enamored fair one was obliged to resort to a peculiar procedure. She had to remove all her clothing in the presence of the witch. Then, lying down, a board was strapped to her loins, upon which a small stove was placed in which the cake was baked. The heat of the stove imparted a perspiring glow to the maiden which gave the bread its finishing touch and flavor. It was then sent, while still warm, to her indifferent lover. Suspecting nothing, he eats ; suddenly the blood rushes to his heart, and ardent love for the devoted bread-maker possesses him. The illustration on the title page of this chapter (taken from an oil painting in the museum at Leipzig) represents such a labor of love. The ingredients evidently possess extraordinary powers, for the lover has already hastened hither and appears at the door in the background.

Stimulating aphrodisiacs were much in use in the earlier centuries of the Middle Ages, since Avicenna says that the plague-like skin-diseases of the ninth century were largely due to these drugs. The " Diasatirion" of Mesue was greatly lauded. Of its properties it is said : " Valet ad erectionem virgæ, multiplicat sperma et desiderium cœundi." Its formula, as given in the Cordic Dispensatory of 1546, is reproduced in the original, as it will hardly bear effective translation :

℞ Secacul. albi et mundi et elixati in decocto Cicerum, quorum prima aqua, in qua decoquebantur, sit effusa, lib. I
>   Testiculorum vulpis unc. VIII
>   Radic. raphani unc. III
>   Rad. Luph. plani unc. II

Terantur hae tres radices posteriores et infundatur super eas lactis bubuli aut ovili tantum, ut lac duos digitos emineat, ajiciendo
>   Olei sesami
>   Butyri recentis non saliti ana unc. IIII

Coquanter cum facilitate usque ad consumptionem lactis et donec omnino remollitae sint radices et habeant justam spissitudinem instar pultis crassioris, nam si aqueum quod in lacte et radicibus est non consumatur, situm contrahit hoc medicamentum. Postea adfunde omnibus hisce praedictis radicibus.
>   Mellis despumati optimi lib. VI
>   Succi Caeparum recentium lib. I β

coque omnia simul ad perfectam decoctionem deinde ab igne depone, et insperge subsequentium specierum minutissimum pulverem.
>   Caudarum Scinccium renibus et semine unc. I
>   Seminis erucae
>   Zingiberis
>   Been albi
>   Been rubei
>   Linguae avis, id est semen fraxini arboris
>   Semanis nasturtii
>   Cinnamomi
>   Piperis longi
>   Seminis Bauciae
>   Seminis napi
>   Pulpae seminis Asparagi maxime recentis ana drach. III
>   Confice cum eis, ultimo vero adjiceantur subsequentia.
>   Pinearum mundatarum lib. I β
>   Fisticorum, id est, Pistaciorum mundatorum unc. X
>   Confice et misce omnia optime et aromatica cum
>   Moschi boni drach. I

The parts of the wolf and skink contained in the formula, indicate that the mixture was not merely intended as a philter, but served on occasions as a remedy for impotence. Signs, offering love-charms and philters, are still to be seen in certain quarters in all large cities, which is evidence that the belief in them has not disappeared from nineteenth century civilization. Love-lorn maidens still wend their way to the drug-store and puzzle a modest clerk with a demand for a "love-powder." If he were to hand them a coal with the advice of Goethe :

> " Take this coal, with it do thou mark
> His arm, his cloak, or his shoulder ;
> In his heart a pang he'll feel,
> But the coal delay not to swallow.

> " Neither of wine nor of water dare drink,
> And this night at your door he will sigh ;
> This coal from a distant land cometh,
> On a funeral pile it hath reposed "—

they would leave his store happy and contented, and try the experiment at once. Numerous domestic methods are still employed to capture and retain the love of others. Many an enamored swain in northern Germany still wears about him for this purpose the blood of a bat, or the heart of a swallow, or he presents his love with an apple that he has carried in his arm-pit for sometime. The efficacy of this last endeavor will be readily accepted by the adherents of Prof. Jaeger's fragrant soul-theory; for, unquestionably, the apple will convey to the adored one some particles of the lover's soul-substance — the "anthropin," whose presence Jaeger easily demonstrated by neuro-analysis with Hipps chronoscope, but which the skeptical chemists continue to call by the names kapron, kaprin and kapryl acids.

In contra-distinction to love-provoking methods, a belief in love-destroying agents is also current among the people. Thus, lovers must not present each other with sharp instruments, such as scissors, knives and needles, lest they " cut love." Many similar notions, current at the present time, might be cited, but these suffice to show how deeply the superstitious notions concerning love-charms are rooted in the human mind. Although the old forms may have fallen away, the " nameless yearning " continually develops new blossoms on the old trunk of superstition. These fallacious notions certainly flourished more luxuriantly in antiquity, when the exuberant imagination and wanton sensuality had not yet been hedged in by a progressive intellectual culture ; still, even in very early days, an occasional warning against the foolish belief in love-charms is heard. Ovid has answered the question, "What is to be thought of love-philters?" entirely in conformity with modern views.

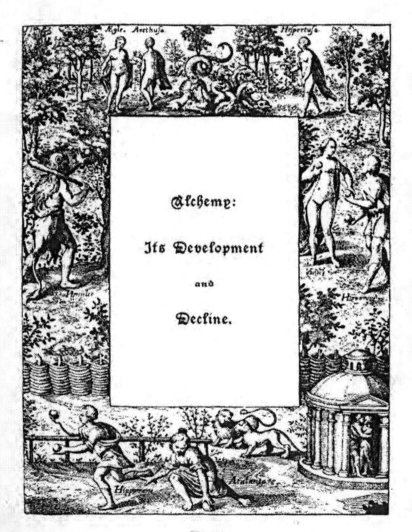

Alchemy:

Its Development

and

Decline.

Fig. 77.

" This natural process, by help of craft then consummate,
Dissolveth the *Elixir* in its unctious humiditie,
Then in *balneo of Mary* together let them circulate,
Like new honey or oil, till they perfectly thickéd be ;
Then will that medicine heal all manner infirmity,
And turn all metal to *Sonne* and *Moone* most perfectly,
Then shall you have both great *Elixir* and *aurum potabile*,
By the grace and will of God, to whom be laud eternally."

*From verses dedicatory of George Ripley " The English Alchemyst
and Canon of Bridlington," addressed to King Edward IV.*

Chapter Eleven.

Alchemy: Its Development and Decline.

RANSMUTATION of the metals, the dream of the alchemists, was abandoned as the wildest of fancies after the discovery of the "elements" now recognized. Spectral analysis has, however, gradually aroused suspicion as to the elementary nature of these elements, so that the present drift of chemical thought is well represented by Mr. Crookes in his address before the British Association for the Advancement of Science, when he approvingly quoted Faraday's words: "To discover a new element is a fine thing, but if you could decompose an element, it would be a discovery indeed worth making. . . . To decompose the metals, then to reform them, to change them from one to another, and to realize the once absurd notion of transmutation, are the problems now given to the chemist for solution."

The labors of the alchemist are better appreciated to-day than they have been for many a decade. The longing for truth which inspires modern science, inspired these old votaries of knowledge in a degree no less ardent and determined.

The dreams of the early alchemists were not always of the sordid type ascribed to them, although the necessity of securing aid from "practical" capitalists led the most sincere to place the "gold-making" side uppermost, just as the scientist of to-day dwells on the "practical" results to secure the aid of plutocrats who are indifferent to the intellectual riches of science. The early alchemists assumed the trade practices and designations so common in the Middle Ages. The disciples were called "fire philosophers" or alchemists, answering to the apprentices of the

(159)

various "crafts" or "mysteries," as all trades were then designated; while the "masters" of the trades became the "adepts" of the alchemist. In consonance with the spirit of the times these "adepts" assumed the owl-like self-satisfied air of concealed wisdom characteristic of those who had reached the height of a "master" of a "mystery" or "craft," and called themselves Φιλόσοφος κατ' εξοχήν.

They are usually thought of as old men, but very brief reflection dispels this notion. Many of the alchemists did their best work before middle age. As alchemy and astrology occupied the place that science does to-day, it was but natural that they should cast a spell over young and enthusiastic minds. Like modern science, alchemy captivated the best and highest circles of society. Venerable monks, renowned physicians, illustrious university professors, mighty statesmen, pious popes and crowned heads were worshippers of alchemy. To it secret hours were given in secluded chambers, behind fire-proof laboratory walls, where they labored day and night at the "Althanor," as the blast-stove of the fire-philosophers was called.

Alchemy is usually traced to the teachings of Hermes Trismegistos, and is hence called the "hermetic" art. It is certain that among the Egyptians chemical studies were a favorite pursuit. The Ayrans and the Chinese were also devoted to them, and at a very early period they had thereby discovered gunpowder. Traces of their teachings and those of the Assyrians, who also paid much attention to these studies, had been left in Central Asia, whence they had been brought to Rome and Greece.

About 400 A. D., the doctrine of the transmutation of metals began to assume prominence. The Greek orator, Themistus Euphrades, in his eighth speech, incidentally speaks of the transmutation of copper into silver and gold as a universally accepted fact. Before the intellectual vigor produced by the contact of the Crusaders with eastern civilization had begun to show itself in Europe, all study was rather quiescent under the turmoil of these periods of "storm and stress." Still such studies were being pursued, for the works of Geber of Seville, written in the ninth century, were too comprehensive to have been the first beginning of the science.

From the time of the Crusades all science received an impetus. Alchemy began to appear prominently in the tenth and the eleventh centuries. The English alchemist, Hortulanus, wrote a Latin paraphrase of the " Tabula Smaragdina," which was said to have originated with Hermes Trismegistos and occupied a conspicuous place in the literature of the alchemist. A translation of the paraphrase is as follows :

THE EMERALD TABLET OF HERMES TRISMEGISTOS.

These are the words of the secret of Hermes, which were written upon the emerald tablet, found in a dark hole where the body of Hermes was buried.

Discoursing as follows :

True it is, and without deceit, certainly and truthfully, that which is below is also above, and that which is above is made like all things by one thing ; his father is Sol and his mother Luna. The wind carried him in its bowels. He was nourished by the earth, which is father of all secrets of the world. His power is absolute. When turned to the earth, it separates the soil from the fire, the subtile from the coarse with great skill. It rises from the earth to the heaven, and returns from the heaven to the earth, and takes upon itself the forces of all that is high and all that is low. Here you have the essence of the world. All poverty and darkness will flee thee, and everything comparable to darkness. Therefore am I called Hermes Trismegistus, possessing the three parts of all philosophy. All this has come to pass as I have described.

Much of the seeming obscurity of alchemical literature was due to the desire to prevent the feudal barons, and other thieves of the period, from seizing on the adepts who thus adopted secrecy as a means of protection. This obscurity long remained in science, but was over-estimated by the popular miscomprehension of the necessity of technical terms. The seeming jargon of the alchemists was not greater than that of the early anatomists, which, while etymologically jargon, has acquired by long-continued usage fixity and clearness of meaning.

The twelfth century witnessed a great development of alchemy The works of Ægidus show that a large literature was being accumulated. Albertus Magnus made extensive studies in the early part of the thirteenth century. By his chemical labors, growing out of the search for the "elixir of life," and the "philosopher's stone," he paved the way for his great successor, Roger Bacon, who attempted to systematize all the knowledge of the time. It was left for the nineteenth century to disentomb his

works from the alcoves of Oxford library, and do his labors
justice. He really placed the study of chemistry on a firm basis.
He enthusiastically pursued the search for the " philosopher's
stone," and the " elixir of life." He introduced gunpowder into
Europe. Though much of his writings seem obscure, yet it has
been aptly said by Gordon, " As even happens in more recent
times, Roger Bacon, in the thirteenth century, concealed much
useful information under that jargon of languages which was so
fashionable in that time." Bacon really led the way in modern
science by insisting on the necessity of experiments in the
acquirement. In all respects he anticipated the inductive philosophy of his famous namesake, Francis Bacon. The inductive
philosophy was the great gift of the alchemists, whose experiments stood out in bold relief for their usefulness as compared
with the " word-juggling " of the Scotists and Thomists, who had
captured the Universities. Raymond Lully wrote several works
on alchemy during this century, which were accepted authorities.
His discussion of the " tabula smaragdina," was the " authority "
on that subject, then one of importance.

The study of alchemy took on such proportions in the fourteenth century that Pope John XXII, who later became a devotee
of the art, condemned the hermetic art as a diabolical deception,
and issued a severe bull to restrict its practice. The sincere
alchemists, however, claimed,—and, judged by the Pope's subsequent career, this claim seems justifiable,—that this bull was issued
against pretenders and swindlers who were befouling the fair
fame of alchemy by their tricks. Certainly the bull was taken
in this sense by priests, for Canon Ripley, of Bridlington, England, in the fourteenth century, wrote an alchemical work, " The
Six Chemical Portals." He explains that alchemists " purposely
use mystic language to discourage the fools, for although we
write primarily for the edification of the disciples of the art, we
also write for the mystification of those owls and bats that can
neither bear the splendor of the sun nor the light of the moon.
On these we practice many cabalistic deceits, which harmonize
with their ill-favored fantasy." Ripley certainly succeeded in
his attempt at mystifying his readers, for his formulas are so
incongruous and contradictory as to be absolutely unintelligible.
This is well illustrated by the following passage :

> " The bird of Hermes is my name,
> Eating my wings to make me tame.
> In the sea withouten lesse
> Standeth the bird is Hermes—
> Fating his wings variable,
> And thereby makete himself more stable.
> When all his feathers be agone
> He standeth still there as a stone ;
> Here is now both white and red,
> And also the stone to quicken the dead ;
> All and some, withouten fable,
> Both hard, and nesh, and malleable.
> Understand now well aright,
> And thanke God of this Light."

Ripley also wrote a " Compound of Alchemy." He was a very assiduous student, and thus describes his experience :

> " Many amalgame did I make,
> Wenyng to fix these to grett avayle,
> And thereto sulphur dyd I take ;
> Tarter, eggs whyts, and the oyl of the snayle,
> But ever of my purpose dyd I fayle ;
> For what for the more and what for the lesse,
> Evermore something wanting there was."

He then gives a long list of ingredients, and concludes :

> " Thus I roastyd and boylyd, as one of Geber's cooks,
> And oft tymes my wynning in the asks I sought ;
> For I was discevyd wyth many false books,
> Whereby untrue thus truly I wrought ;
> But all such experiments avayled me nought ;
> But brought me in danger and in combraunce,
> By losse of my goods and other grevaunce."

The swindling alchemist early made his appearance, and was satirized by Chaucer in his " Canterbury Tales."

> " The priest him busieth, all that ever he can
> To don as this Chanoun, this cursed man,
> Commandeth him, and fast blew the fire.
> For to come to the effect of his desire ;
> And this Chanoun right in the meanwhile
> All ready was this priest eft to beguile,
> And for a countenance in his hand bare
> An hollow stick (take, keep, and beware),
> In the end of which an ounce, and no more,
> Of silver limaille put was as before ;

"Was in his coal, and stopped with wax well
For to keep in his limaille every del.
And while this priest was in his business
This Chanoun with his stick gave him dress,
To him anon, and his powder cast in,
As he did erst (the devil out of his skin)
Him turn, I pray to God, for his falsehede),
For he was ever false in thought and deed,
And with his stick above the crosslet,
That was ordained with that false get,
He stirreth the coals, til relenten gan
The wax again the fire as every man
But he a fool be, wot well it wote need,
And all that in the stick was out yede ;
And in the crosslet hastily it fell."

Norton was an active "adept" in the fifteenth century. His "Ordinal," published in 1477, opens thus :

" Maistryeful, merveilous, and archaimaistrye
Is the tincture of holy alkimy.
A wonderful science, secrete philosophie ;
A singular gift and grace of the Almightie,
Which never was found by the labour of mann ;
But by teaching or revelacion begann.
It was never for money sold or bought,
By any mann which for it has sought,
But given to an able mann by grace,
Wrought with great cost, by long laisir and space,
It helpeth a man when he hath neede ;
It voideth vain glory, hope and also dreade ;
It voideth ambitiousness, extortion and excesse ;
It fenceth adversity that she doe not oppresse."

Italy swarmed with alchemists in the fifteenth century. The Senate of Venice, in 1468, passed stringent laws prohibiting them from further pursuing their vocation. The Nuremburg Senate, in 1493, enacted laws for suppressing alchemy. "For many people have, by its practice, not only been ruined in purse, but have also experienced irreparable injury to their moral nature, and have consequently fallen into disgrace."

In the reign of Henry VI of England, an act was passed which ordains "That no one shall henceforth multiply gold or silver, nor use the craft of multiplication, because many persons by color of this multiplication make false money, to the great deceit of the King, and the injury of the people."

One of the greatest alchemists of the fifteenth century was Basil Valentine, to whom is due the discovery of antimony. The following instructions to his disciples show that he was a true scientist :

First, therefore, the name of God ought to be called on religiously with a pure heart and sound conscience, without ambition, hypocrisy, and other abuses, such as are pride, arrogance, disdain, worldly boasting, and oppression of our neighbors, and other enormities of that kind, all of which are to be totally eradicated out of the heart. . . . . Whosoever, therefore, hath resolved within himself to seek the top of terrestrials, that is, the knowledge of the good lodging in every creature lying dormant, or covered in stones, herbs, roots, seeds, living creatures, plants, minerals, metals, and the like, let him cast behind him all worldly cares, and other appurtenances, and expect release with his whole heart by humble prayer, and his hope shall not fail. Men who began and pursued their life-long toil in this spirit are not to be spoken of without great respect.

Emperor Rudolph II, in the sixteenth century, was an ardent student of alchemy. He invited alchemists from far and near to his court. After his death, in 1612, 8,400 pounds of gold, and 6,000 pounds of silver, cast in earthen-pots, were found among his effects, which led to the belief that Rudolph II had been an adept.

Among the leaders of the " Reformation," alchemy acquired friends. Luther says : " The art of Alchemy is, in truth and in fact, the philosophy of the wise. I think highly of it, not only for its inherent virtues and usefulness in the distilling and subliming of metals, herbs and waters, but also for its grand and beautiful similitude to the resurrection of the dead on the day of judgment." The swindling type of alchemist became very frequent in the sixteenth century, and fell under the ridicule of Ben Jonson. The real scientist continued his studies, discoveries of value followed, and a useful foundation was laid for the advances made in the next century. The publication of the works of Francis Bacon stimulated the spirit of philosophical research. The growing science of astronomy dealt the astrological part of alchemy a severe blow, and injured it in the estimation of the learned, who had begun to separate the chaff from the wheat.

Evidences of a growing science of chemistry are discernible in the sixteenth century. In 1654 an alchemist's society was formed at Nuremburg, with the preacher Daniel Wulfel at its head, which remained in existence until 1694. In 1666 the great philosopher, G. W. Leibnitz, received the degree of doctor of laws at Altdorf, and visited savants of Nuremburg, where he heard of this society of learned men, who were secretly endeavoring, by chemical experiments, to discover the "philosopher's stone."

Leibnitz was of an inquisitive turn of mind, and determined to gain an insight into chemistry. To secure admission into this august circle he devised a clever scheme. He read a number of profound chemical works, and collated all obscure words and sentences. From these he framed an incomprehensible letter, which he sent to the priest, with a petition for admission to the secret society. The priest, on reading the letter, concluded that Leibnitz must be an "adept," and not only introduced him into the laboratory, but begged him to accept a salaried position as secretary, which he did. Leibnitz left Nuremberg in 1667, and consequently did not hold this office for a great length of time. Traces of his alchemical studies are evident in his correspondence concerning Newton.

The influence of Francis Bacon showed itself in the scientific study of alchemy in England during the seventeenth century. The "Royal Society" was formed under the protectorate of Cromwell, and its effects were visible in the subsequent reign. King Charles II, Prince Rupert (of whose chemical studies "Prince Rupert's drop" preserves the memory), the Duke of Buckingham, merchants, and even poets, ardently devoted themselves to the labors of the laboratory. Dryden, in his "Annus Mirabilis," glowingly describes the advances made and prophesies others. The Marquis of Worcester devises a rude steam engine as a result of his studies, and pronounces it a "forcible instrument of propulsion." Traces of the infant science of agricultural chemistry are found at this time as a result of the stimulus then given to chemistry. Nor was the hypothesis of the transmutation of metals entirely lost sight of in these studies. Newton spent many hours in his laboratory working at this problem. In his letters to Boyle there are constant references to this pursuit, and to a mysterious red earth needed to complete the transmutation. Elias Ashmole, the founder of the Ashmolean Museum, took occasion to collate the works of the old alchemists in his rare book, published in 1652, the "Theatrum Chemicum Britannicum." These labors point to a growing interest in alchemic literature. In his preface Ashmole says of himself:

I must profess I know enough to hold my tongue, but not enough to speak,—and the no less real than miraculous fruits I have found in my diligent inquiry into this arcana, lead me on to such degrees of admiration they command silence, and force me to loose my tongue. Howbeit there are few stocks that are fitted to inoculate the grafts of science upon ; they are mysteries uncommunicable to all but adepts, and those that have been devoted from their cradle to serve and wait at this altar—and they, perhaps, were, with St. Paul, caught up into Paradise, and as he heard unspeakable words—so they wrought impossible works.

Frequent attempts were made to explain and amplify the principles laid down in alchemical works, by the introduction of picturesque, obscure and mystical circumlocutions. Poetry, music and art were frequently pressed into service. Alchemy is expounded by aid of these agents in the " Atalanta fugiens, hoc est emblemata nova de secretis naturæ chymica. Authore Michaele Majero. Oppenheimii, 1618," from which Fig. 77, on the title-page of this chapter is taken. This illustration is intended to demonstrate the dangers of the search for the " philosopher's stone," which is compared to the wooing of the swift-footed, beautiful Bœotian, Atalanta. According to the myth, she stipulated that every suitor must run a race with her, in which he was given a start. In case she did not overtake him, she was to be his wife ; otherwise he was to die. Many suitors had perished in this manner, when Hippomenes, by the aid of Aphrodite, outwitted Atalanta. The goddess gave him golden apples, which he dropped in the path of his pursuer. Atalanta lost so much time picking these up, that Hippomenes reached the goal first. He forgot to thank the kind goddess, who, in revenge, excited him to such vehement manifestations of love, that he embraced his bride in the temple of Zeus. To punish this desecration, the lovers were turned into lions. The garden of the Hesperides is included in this pictorial rendering of the Atalanta legend. In this garden the three daughters of night and the hundred-headed cerberus watched the golden apples, which Hera had received as a present from Gœa at the time of her marriage with Zeus. Hercules secured these apples and brought them to Eurystheus, who returned them to him. Hercules then presented them to Athena, who returned them to the gardens of the Hesperides. Every

precept in this book appears as an epigram, with notes for a
choral melody. A German translation of the verse is given, and
with it a copper plate, designed as an allegorical explanation, of
the precepts it was designed to inculcate. Each chapter winds
up with a verbose supplementary explanation in Latin. Figures
9 and 10, from this work, refer to the alchemistic precepts

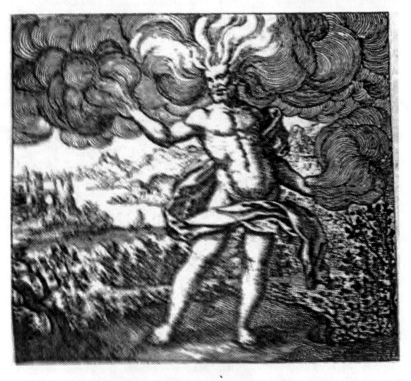

inculcate. The figure illus-
trates its powers and
subjects to the earth. The
following verse

right side that
. . . in a great

The notes on following page (Fig. 80) comprise the melody of the Latin epigram. This poetico-musico pictorial explanation rather conduces to obscurity than to facilitate a solution of the problem.

The influence which astrology exerted on the figurative writings of the alchemists is unmistakeable. Thus there was

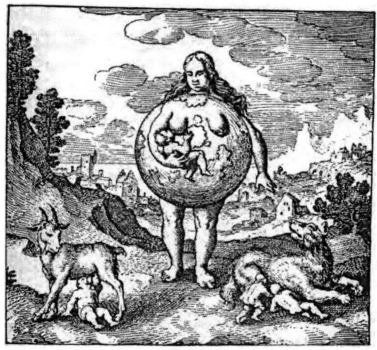

Fig. 79.

supposed to be a close conformity between the seven known metals and the seven so-called planets. This belief was carried into modern chemistry. Each metal was named after the planet upon which it was nominally dependent. Gold was called the sun; silver, the moon; iron, mars; mercury, mercury; tin, jupiter; copper, venus; and lead, saturn. According to the alchemists no planet could suffer a modification without awakening the sympathy of the corresponding metal. This sympathy was, according to astrologico-alchemistic views, transmitted by infinitely minute bodies, which proceeded from the planets and metals. These molecules were so constructed that they could readily enter the pores of the corresponding planet or metal, but never into those of a foreign body. If by chance they came in contact with a foreign body they would not be retained or in any event could not serve as nourishment. Each of the seven

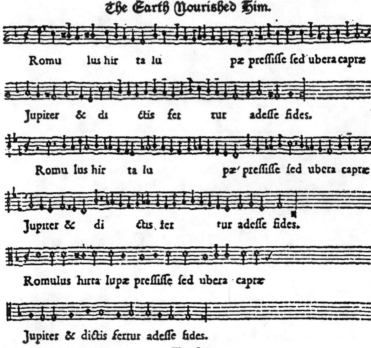

Fig. 80.

planets had its day of the week on which it manifested its influence over its particular metal. To be successful all work with gold must be begun on Sunday; with silver, on Monday; with iron, on Tuesday, etc. All metals were supposed to contain mercury and sulphur. These designations, however, were not those of the substances now known by these names, but others of an entirely different character, of the nature of which the alchemists themselves had no clear conception. Therefore, they spoke of them allegorically, or in respect to their activity.

Sulphur (Sulphur philosophorum) was of an almost spiritual nature; it was the light, the fire and the combustible matter thought to be inherent in all bodies,—the phlogiston of early chemistry. It was the male element, and contained the "Punctum seminale activum" needed in the evolution of new bodies and substances. Alchemistic writers refer to it by many different names,—"House of the Spirit," "Father," "Elementary Fire," "Magical Steel," "Elementary Oil," "Elementary Sulphurous-

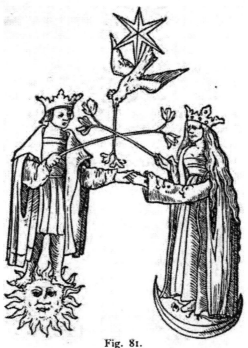

Fig. 81.

ness," "Cadmi-blood," "Adamic-earth," "Heart of Saturn," etc. The female element required to evolve a new body was "Mercurius"; upon it the male, "Sulphur," by intimate contact, impressed the germ of the object to be evolved.

"Mercury," the connecting link between spirit and body, also known as Encheiresis naturæ, was present in the three realms of nature. In the mineral kingdom it was "mineral moisture." In the animal kingdom, "elementary moisture," upon which depended blood and life ; in the plant kingdom, the force or "spiritus mundi," which promoted the growth of the plants. By the old fire philosophers it was called "a water which does not moisten the hands," a "dry moisture" or the "corporeal spirit."

This peculiar "sulphur" and the "mercury," either separately or combined in an hermaphrodite being, were called the "lapis philosophorum," which was also known as the "universal menstruum," the "great magister," the "red tincture," the "secret elixir," the "quinta essentia," etc. The philosopher's stone is pictured by the alchemists as an hermaphrodite being; "sulphur" as the king or sun, and "mercury" as the queen or moon. Fig. 81 (a wood cut from the "Rosarium Philosophorum," printed by Cyriacus Jacobus, at Frankfurt, in 1550), shows the father and the mother of the hermaphrodite stone, in the act of uniting. The stone itself is allegorically represented in figure 82. To indicate the enigmatical character of this being, it is surrounded by the animals that took part, according to the allegory, in the formation of the stone. In honor of the latter, the following verse is appended to this picture, called the "Ænigma Regis."

> " Here a king is born indeed,
>   None can boast of nobler breed ;
>   Formed he was by art or nature,
>   His birth he owes to no known creature.
>   Of philosophers he is the son,
>   Of their power an incarnate one ;
>   Health and life he freely gave,
>   And every wish that man may crave ;
>   Silver, gold and gems so rare,
>   Youth and strength and all that's fair ;
>   From him flee anger, grief and pains,
>   Whoe'er from God this gift obtains.

Thus, the philosopher's stone, not only changed metals into gold, but, according to some, could change any substance into gold, cure all diseases, and control, renew and rejuvenate animal life.

Every alchemist goes into raptures over the "quinta essentia," the soul of the four elements. The alchemists, Artephius and Cagliostro, claimed to have lived over one thousand years by the aid of this elixir. Ripley lauds its medicinal virtues in a rapturous style, calling it the greatest medicine in the world. He declares " It is the true tree of life, which gratifies all desires of the person possessing it. It rejuvenates, retards old age, strengthens and restores health. It will not only produce a new growth of hair, but, properly applied, will prevent hair from turning

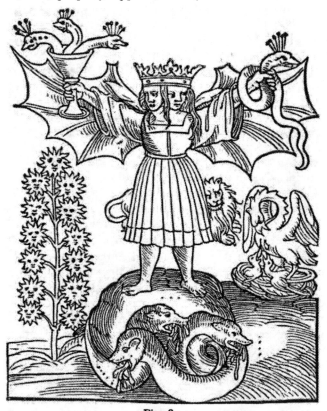

Fig. 82.

REPRESENTATION OF THE FORMATION OF THE HERMAPHRODITE STONE.

gray." The "quinta essentia," which was sold at a high price under the name of "aurum potabile," was, for the most part, golden-yellow vegetable tinctures of about the same value as the "infallible hair restorers " of the barber.

Diverse methods were adopted to secure the great desideratum. Some alchemists sought the philosopher's stone in

honey, manna, sugar or wine; others in vegetables, like rose-
mary and marquory, or in gums, blood, urine or excrements.
Some sought it in may-dew and rainwater. Astrologists went to
the extent of imprisoning the sun's rays, and attempting to cal-
cine and powder them. The rays were supposed to consist of
pure golden sparks, which contained the seed of gold. The dead
were not allowed to rest in the grave. From their decaying
bodies saltpetre was extracted, which was regarded as the soul
of the philosopher's stone,—the " true microcosm."

Other fire philosophers considered various kinds of earth; for
example, marl, as the " chaos " from which God made the world,
and sought for the seed of all things, the " panspermion," in the
earth itself. This seed was thought to be a formless, peculiar
being, which possessed the power to create all things, gold being
the most distinguished.

Opposed to these theories was a party headed by Raymond
Lully and Basil Valentine, who boldly asserted that the light of
Nature was but the light of an *ignis fatuus* or glow-worm. This
party had for the cardinal principle in their philosophy, " Omne
simile suum simile," and consequently sought the seed of gold in
gold itself. They considered other metals as merely furnishing
a fruitful soil in which the gold seed was sown, and which would,
by a process of interstitial displacement, develop and grow like
a plant. For purposes of fructification, it was thought essential
to steep golden seed in its own moisture. This gold-like
moisture, called " metallic water," was no doubt mercury. It
was not, however, the common marketable article, " but only
such as had been skillfully extracted from the objects in which
it is found in nature. The 'Mercurius philosophorum' is not
found on the face of the earth, but, as Philaletha says, ' is the
son that is prepared by us.'" The purification of mercury,
essential to its union with gold to form the philosopher's stone,
is given much attention in alchemistic literature. Numerous formulas for mercurial compounds are given, from which purified
mercury can be obtained. The " Hermetic Philosophy " of John
d'Espagnet, gives a formula for preparing mild mercury chloride,
which does not materially differ from the modern process. The
descriptive part, however, is so characteristic of the times, that
it merits reproduction here :

" The eagle and the lion, after being thoroughly cleansed, are put together in a transparent reservoir. This is tightly closed, so that their breath cannot escape, or air enter from without. The eagle will dismember and eat the lion : and when his stomach is swollen, and he has become dropsical, he will, by a wonderful transformation, be changed into a coal-black raven, which will gradually spread its feathers and begin to fly, and shake water from the clouds until he has become wet several times, lost his feathers, and finally fallen to the bottom, when he will be changed into a snow-white swan."

The " eagle " is the volatile mercury, which, combined with the " lion," or mercuric chloride, produces the black compound, "the raven," from which the mild mercury chloride, the white swan, is made by sublimation from a glass retort, to which an air-tight receptacle has been adjusted, after the surplus of mercury, here called " water," has become separated. The purification and sublimation of mercury was repeated seven times. The seed gold had to be cleansed an equal number of times before it was amalgamated. The gold was to battle with the seven eagles of the philosophical " arsenic," and then unite itself with the two doves of Diana. The eagles indicate the mercurial volatility of the metal used, called " philosophical arsenic " (properly speaking, antimony), with which the gold was to be melted seven times. This is an old method for purifying gold. By the heating process the foreign metals and admixtures which frequently accompany the gold are slaked with the antimony and a little saltpetre, whilst the pure gold, the king of metals, subsides to the bottom of the crucible.

" But before the gold is mixed with its water it must be reduced to the finest powder possible or it will withstand solution." To reduce gold to this fine powder it was, according to an old formula, melted with two parts of silver, called by the alchemists, the two doves from Diana's forest, that is, the metallic kingdom, and this alloy was treated with nitric acid. The silver was dissolved by the acid, and the gold remained undissolved in the acid as a very fine powder, although still somewhat contaminated by small particles of silver. This gold powder, which the alchemists believed to be absolutely pure, readily united with mercury under the influence of a gentle heat, and it was this mixture which represented the " true hermaphrodite," whose male generic element descended from the most perfect of metals, and whose female force is a delicate mineral whiteness. It was supposed to contain the egg from which the "philosopher's stone" was developed.

To this end a glass retort was filled with the amalgam, placed in a nest-like contrivance on a stove, and subjected to a gentle, even heat for nearly a year, "because it also takes a kernel of wheat that length of time to develop and produce new kernels." The "stone" was not to be disturbed during this process of development, as its incipient vitality might thus be easily destroyed. During the first three months, its embryonic period, it was kept at an animal temperature. At the end of this time it had changed into white "magisterium," and could change baser metals into silver. The temperature was then gradually raised in five stages of variable duration, during which time the stone changed color like a chameleon. From the original black raven, which had changed into a white dove, a Tyrian purple color was to result, which was the true "philosopher's stone." "Projection" (sprinkling it on molten metal), would change a metal into gold. Ripley says that one grain could change one hundred ounces of mercury into the so-called red tincture, and calculates that with this exactly 119,010⅛ pounds of mercury could be changed into gold.

Raymond Lully, during his sojourn in London, is said to have transformed 50,000 pounds of mercury into gold for King Edward III, from which the first rose-nobles were coined. The credibility of this story, gravely related by the Abbe Cremer, receives a severe shock, when, in spite of this abundant supply of gold, King Edward III is forced to increase the taxes to carry on his war against France, and to coin money from his own and the queen's crown, and from the gold vessels of churches and cloisters.

Koehler, in 1744, related in his numismatical work, that the Emperor Frederic III, although not a disciple of alchemy, changed, on January 15, 1648, at Prague, three pounds of mercury into two and one-half pounds of gold by means of one grain of a red powder, given him by a man named Richthausen. He created this man a Baron of Chaos, and from the gold a medal was made which bore an inscription referring to the artificial origin of the gold. This medal was long preserved in the Vienna Treasury.

Urban Hjœrne, a renowned chemist of his day, reports a

similar case of transformation from Sweden. The Saxon lieu-
tenant, Paykull, was taken prisoner by Charles XII, at Warsau,
in 1705, and condemned to death. He promised to make one
million dollars worth of gold each year, if his life were spared.
Paykull changed lead into gold by means of a tincture, rendered
fire-proof by the addition of antimony, sulphur and saltpetre. In
the presence of Hamilton, the master of ordnance, Paykull, with
an ounce of this mixture, changed six ounces of lead into gold.
To make a counter-test, Hamilton mixed the powders at home.
Paykull next day added some of the tincture, and the whole was
melted together with a quantity of lead. Gold to the value of
one hundred and forty-seven ducats was secured. Out of this
gold medals of two-ducat weight were coined, and inscribed as
follows : " Hoc aurum arte chemica conflavit Holmiæ, 1706.
O. A. v. Paykull." Paykull, despite his skill, was executed.

The gold-makers, though for the most part, generous and in-
dustrious, devoting themselves to the enrichment of others, rather
than themselves, frequently met a cruel fate. George Honauer
promised to transform thirty-six hundred weight of iron into
gold for the Prince of Wirtemburg. The prince detected a boy,
who had been concealed in the laboratory, in the act of putting
gold into the crucible. He thereupon ordered a gallows to be
constructed of iron from which the false gold-maker was hung
in 1597. In 1606 a gold-maker, named Andreas von Muehlen-
dorf, was hung at Stuttgart on this same gallows, which gained
further repute in 1738, by its services in the execution of minister
Joseph Suess, who knew, without the aid of the " hermetic art,"
better than " adepts," how to make gold.

Chr. Wm. Krohnemann, in 1677, entered the service of the
Marquis of Brandenburg, with the rank of colonel. In a short
time he won a high reputation as a gold-maker, and was rapidly
promoted to the directorship of the mint and mines. From gold
ostensibly made by Krohnemann, seven different medals were
coined, which are pictured and described in the "Book of Odd
Historical Coins," published in 1771. Figure 83, taken from this
book, represents the first, the largest and rarest specimen in
the Krohnemann numismatic cabinet. On the obverse is a
fettered Mercury, who holds in his hand a staff, terminating in a
sun, emblematic of gold. The whole figure serves as an alchem-

istic symbol. It is surrounded by a Latin dedicatory inscription to "Margrave Christian Ernst, 1677." The reverse bears a Latin inscription to the following effect: "Let it be known to all, that

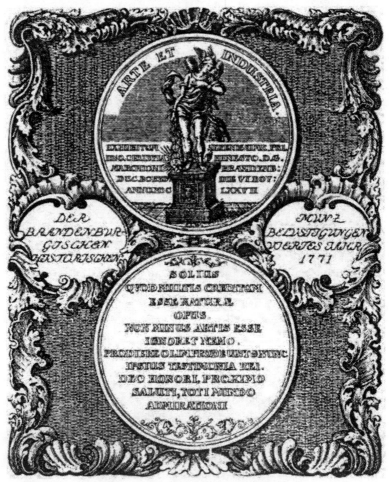

Fig. 83.

ALCHEMISTIC GOLD COINS.

what by many is supposed to be the work of nature only, can also be accomplished by art. This product is witness thereof, to the honor of God, for the well-being of thy neighbor and the

admiration of the wide world." The last coin made by Krohnemann was a small medal dedicated to Margravess Sophia Louise,
of Brandenburg, in 1681. After this medal had been coined,
Krohnemann was suspected of deception, and imprisoned in
1681, in the Plassenburg citadel. He continued his experiments
until 1686, when he escaped. He was recaptured, tried and
found guilty of having abstracted gold and silver ware from the
Margrave's treasury, for use in his deception. As it was also
proven that he unlawfully cohabited with his jaileress, he was
condemned to be hanged for fraud, theft and adultery. In the
course of the trial it was demonstrated that Krohnemann had
worked according to a formula in general use among the alchemists of his day. Berzelius, in his text-book, thus describes it :

" Mercury, verdigris, vitriol and salt are digested with strong vinegar in an
iron-pot, and stirred with an iron-rod until the mass takes on the consistency of
butter. The remaining liquid, which is an amalgam of copper, is pressed
through leather, and then put into a crucible with even parts of curcuma and
tutia, whereupon the crucible is heated by a blast. The curcuma reduces the
tutia, which is an impure oxide of zinc, and the copper in the amalgam unites
with the zinc to form brass. Krohnemann surreptitiously added gold ; hence
his product was an alloy of copper, gold and zinc."

A quack named Daniel supplied Italian apothecaries with a
wonderful gold-powder called "Usufur." Pretending that the
art of compounding this usufur with other drugs was a mystery
known only to himself, he directed his patients not to permit the
apothecaries to mix the ingredients of his prescriptions, but to
buy them (including the usufur), and bring them to him for compounding. His "art" consisted in compounding the drugs, but
omitting the golden "usufur," in which manner he succeeded in
having restored to him the gold-powder, which he had previously sold at a high price. The powder soon became famous
under the shrewd practices of the quack, who finally offered to
teach Duke Cosmos II, of Florence, the art of making gold. He
asked the duke himself to buy the "usufur" at a drug-store, and
with this the experiment was of course a success. After the
duke had repeatedly succeeded in making gold according to
directions, he paid Daniel 20,000 ducats, who thereupon fled
beyond the border to France, whence he wrote the duke how he
had been victimized.

Alchemy was practiced at the Saxon court during the reign

of Prince August (1553 to 1586), who had the reputation of an
"adept." One of his collaborators, David Benter, after many
trials, failed to produce gold, whereupon he was imprisoned on
the strength of an opinion rendered by the highest court of
justice at Leipzig. Having written on the walls of his cell,
"Caged cats catch no mice ;" and having renewed his promises,
he was released to renew his experiments. He lost faith in his
ability to prove his pretensions, and poisoned himself, which
probably saved him the fate of John Hector von Kletten-
berg, a Saxon alchemist, decapitated in 1620. Count Cajetan,
in 1705, in the presence of Frederic I of Prussia, changed, by
means of his red tincture, one pound of mercury into gold. He
did not keep his promise of making six million dollars of gold in
six weeks, and in 1709 was hanged, draped in gold leaf, which
became the customary method of dealing with alchemists.

The numerous deceptions practiced in connection with the
philosopher's stone, explain the solemn oaths of witnesses of
known integrity, whose testimony would otherwise be unimpeach-
able, but who were in reality themselves duped and deceived.
Contemporaneous writers did not fail to remonstrate against
alchemistic pretensions, and vigorously expose their fallacy. The
enlightened Parisian apothecary, Nicol. Lemery, in his " Cours
de Chimie," calls alchemy satirically, " Ars sine arte, cujus prin-
cipium mentiri, medium laborare et finis mendicare."—" An art-
less art, whose beginning is a lie, whose middle is work, and
whose end is poverty."

Although the old fire-philosophers failed to realize their ulti-
mate hope, their labors were not entirely in vain. The belief in
the feasibility of metal transmutation stimulated wide research
in the domain of nature. The search for the philosopher's
stone revealed truths which form the basis of modern chemistry, which has been infinitely more successful than its parent,
alchemy, in filling with gold the coffers of its disciples. For
paving the way to this result, a debt of gratitude is due to
alchemy. In spite of the numerous deceptions practiced by the
impostors among its disciples, sympathy must be felt with the
sincere alchemists in contemplating their indomitable courage
and patience in the presence of centuries of repeated failures
and disappointments. Lord Bacon says :

"The alchemist goes on with an eternal hope, and where his matters succeed not, lays the blame upon his own errors, and accuses himself as having not sufficiently understood either the terms of his art, or his author ; whence he either hearkens out for traditions and auricular whispers, or else fancies he made some mistake as to the exact quantity of the ingredients, or nicety of the experiment ; and thus repeats the operation without end. If, in the meantime, among all the chances of experiments, he throws any which appear either new or useful, he feeds his mind with these as so many earnests ; boasts and extols them above measure ; and conceives great hopes of what is behind. ' Now the marriage is consummated !' he exclaims ; the 'philosopher's stone is found,' only to be again deceived. To-day, transported with wild ecstacy ; to-morrow, dejected by utter despair. Thus oscillating, he plodded through life, until kind death stepped in to put an end to his weird fancies." His epitaph was written by Spenser, and none could be more to the point :

> "To lose good days that might be better spent,
> To waste long nights in pensive discontent ;
> To spend to-day, to put back to-morrow ;
> To feed on hope, to pine with fear and sorrow ;
> To fret his soul with crosses and with cares,
> To eat his heart through comfortless despairs :
> Unhappy wight ! born to disastrous end,
> That did his life in tedious tendance spend."

Early in the eighteenth century the passion for making gold still prevailed ; but, at the close of the century it lost ground fast, and was swept away by the new chemistry, which regarded the metals as elements. Concerning one of the last true believers in the "hermetic art," Peter Woulfe, Mr. Brande* says : "He occupied chambers in Barnard's inn, while residing in London, and usually spent the summer in Paris. His rooms, which were extensive, were so filled with furnaces and apparatus, that it was difficult to reach his fireside. A friend told me that he once put down his hat, and never could find it again, such was the confusion of boxes, packages and parcels that lay about the chamber. His breakfast hour was four in the morning ; a few of his select friends were occasionally invited to this repast, to whom a secret

*Quarterly Review, Vol. XXVI.

signal was given, by which they gained entrance. He had long
vainly searched for the elixir, and attributed his repeated failures
to the want of due preparation by pious and charitable acts. I
understand that some of his apparatus is still extant, upon which
are supplications for success, and for the welfare of adepts.
Whenever he wished to break an acquaintance, or felt himself
offended, he resented the supposed injury by sending a present
to the offender, and never seeing him afterward. These presents
were sometimes of a curious description, and consisted usually
of some expensive chemical product or preparation. .He had an
heroic remedy for illness ; when he felt himself seriously indis-
posed, he took a place in the Edinburgh mail, and, having reached
that city, immediately came back in the returning coach to London. A cold taken on one of these expeditions, terminated in
an inflammation of the lungs, of which he died in 1805.

' "About the same time another solitary adept starved in London. He was an editor of an evening journal, and expected to
compound the 'alcahest,' if he could only keep his materials
digested in a lamp-furnace for seven years. The lamp burnt
brightly for six years, eleven months, and some odd days, then
unluckily it went out. Why it went out the adept could never
guess; but he was certain that if the flame would only have
burnt to the end of the septennary cycle, his experiment must
have succeeded."

The race of alchemists of the type of Krohnemann is not
entirely extinct, for, in 1880, an American called Wise, duped a
member of the Rohan family, and a collateral descendant of the
"necklace cardinal," whom Cagliostro so deceived, by pretending to make gold. The first specimen made in Rohan's presence
was tested and proved pure. Rohan was not permitted to be
present at the process of "projection." Wise got a considerable
sum from Rohan, and then decamped.

LATER ALCHEMISTIC SYMBOLS.

From the primitive symbolism of alchemy grew up the complicated system seen in the following table, which gave way in its turn to the chemical symbolism of to-day:

✝	Acetum	Vinegar.
✢	" destillatum	Distilled Vinegar.
△	Aer	Air.
⊕	Aerugo.............................	Greenspar.
○	Alumen.............................	Alum.
⊖	Ammoniac..........................	Ammoniac.
♁	Antimonium	Antimony.
▽	Aqua	Water.
℣	Aqua fortis	Nitric Ac'd.
℞	" Regis.......................	Nitro Hydrochloric Acid.
⛰	Arena..............................	Sand.
☽	Argentum	Silver.
⚭	Arsenic	Arsenic.
∞	Auripigmentum	Orpiment.
○	Aurum..............................	Gold.
♉	Baryta	Barium.
♄	Bismuthum	Bismuth.
⏢	Borax..............................	Borax.
♄	Calcium............................	Calcium.
≋	Camphora	Camphor.
☺	Caput Mortuum	Skull.
♋	Cancer	Crab.
♒	Carbo..............................	Charcoal.
♄	Cineres Clavellati	Potash.
⊔	Cinis..............................	Ash.
♅	Cinnabaris.........................	Cinnabar.
☒	Crystalli..........................	Crystal.
♀	Cuprum, Venus.....................	Copper.
♃	Detur	Let it be given.
♃	Detur Signetur....................	Let it be given and write.
♂	Dies	Day.
♂	Ferrum............................	Iron.
♄	Herba	Herb.
✕	Hora..............................	Hour.

△	Ignes	Fire.
🜃	Lapis	Stone.
⚶	Magnesi	Magnesia.
⊠	Menstruum	Menstruum.
☿	Mercurius	Mercury.
MR	Mistura	Mixture.
⦶	Nitrum	Saltpetre.
⚲	Nox	Night.
∞	Oleum Ætherum	Ethereal Oil.
⊖⊖	Oxymel.	Oxymel.
⚴	Phosphorus	Phosphorus.
☽☉	Platinum	Platinum.
♄	Plumbum	Lead.
≂	Præcipitatum	Precipitate.
PP	Præparare	Prepare Powders.
♁♀	Pulv. Pulvis	Powder.
Ƴ	Regulus	Regulus.
σ	Retorta	Retort.
⊖	Sal	Salt.
⊖X⊖X	Sal Ammoniacum	Sal Ammoniac.
⊝	Sal Medium	Middle Salt.
O♀	Sal Tartari	Cream of Tartar.
▭	Sapo	Soap.
ß	Semis	Half.
~	Spiritus	Spirit.
VV	Spirit Vini	Alcohol.
VR	" " Rectificatus	Rectified Alcohol.
VRff	" " Rectificatissumus	Double Rectified Alcohol.
♃	Stannum	Tin.
≏	Sublimare	Sublime.
🜍	Sulphur	Sulphur.
♀	Tartarus	Tartar.
∀	Terre	Earth.
∀	Terra Foliata	Leaf Earth.
℞	Tinctura	Tincture.
⊡	Urina	Urine.
⊕	Vitriolum	Vitriol.
XX	Vitrum	Glass.
Λ	Volatile	Volatile.
♁	Zincum	Zinc.

Printed in the United States
95999LV00002BA/10/A

9 781432 523930